THE WHIC
GUIDE T
BIRTH CON

THE WHICH? GUIDE TO BIRTH CONTROL

Penny Kane

Published by Consumers' Association and Hodder & Stoughton

Acknowledgements

Many people contributed ideas and knowledge to this book. Among them were the staff of the Family Planning Association – in particular Toni Belfield and Romie Goodchild – and the International Planned Parenthood Federation, especially Ronald Kleinman. Others include Isobel Allan, Caspar Brook, Walli Bounds, Dilys Cossey, Elphis Christopher, Liz Deeds, Helene Grahame, John Guillebaud, Philip Kestelman, David Paintin, Rodney Schearman, Gordon Snow and Pramilla Senanayake. None of them, of course, is responsible for the views expressed here.

Neither is Robert Snowden, to whom particular gratitude is due both for his pioneering work on contraception as a consumer issue, and for the time and effort he gave to this book, right from the earliest planning stage.

Dr Malcolm Potts and his team thought up the idea of presenting the points of intervention in fertility as a Y diagram. We have adapted their original concept a little, but are grateful for that idea.

Published in Great Britain by
Consumers' Association
14 Buckingham Street, London WC2N 6DS
and Hodder & Stoughton Limited
47 Bedford Square, London WC1B 3DP

Written by Penny Kane
Edited by Sarah Wright
Designed by Bridget Morley and Patrick Nugent
Illustrated by Russell Barnett; diagrams by Nick Harris
Cartoon reproduced by permission of Punch

ISBN 0 340 32232 2

Filmset in Apollo by
Filmtype Services Limited,
Scarborough, North Yorkshire.

Contents

Preface

Back in 1963, when *Which?* published its first contraceptive supplement, 'it was difficult to get good, straightforward information and advice about contraception. It wasn't always respectable even to ask. And the contraceptives around at that time were by no means all effective – with no-one to tell you which were and which weren't.' At that time, local authorities were not even empowered to give information to the unmarried; the Family Planning Association restricted its services to married couples, or to those engaged and about to be married. The Pill was new and the IUD little used. *Which?* tested hundreds of brands of chemicals and condoms and found that many were of poor quality.

Eleven years later, after the contraceptives supplement had gone through three editions and been bought by a quarter of a million people, it was replaced by *Sex With Health – The Which? Guide to Contraceptives, Abortion and Sex-related Diseases*. Contraception, it said, 'has at last become a respectable and serious part of public health'. The Government had decided to bring family planning into the National Health Service and the contraceptives available had improved.

Yet the fact that *Which?* included a section on sex-related diseases was an indication of residual embarrassment about the subject. During the 1970s, almost every publication about birth control had such a section: it was a kind of Awful Warning which conferred respectability on an otherwise dubious area. Sexually transmitted diseases, though, are to do with sex rather than contraception.

Which? hoped that people did not need to buy a quarter of a million copies of *Sex With Health* over the next ten years. 'It shouldn't take until 1984 to solve the relatively simple public health problems that sex brings.'

So why are we now producing yet another Guide?

The first answer is that, as the range of contraceptives available has been more intensively tested and researched, more and more information about it has become available. Some of the results are helpful, others alarming; many seem contradictory or confusing. Many of the methods described in *Sex with Health* have been adapted or refined. Among the profusion of low-dose Pills, mini-Pills, progestagen-only Pills, triphasic Pills and sequential Pills, for example, it is not easy to pick one's way.

So people continue to ask for a new edition of the Guide, to explain clearly and simply what all these various contraceptives are and how they differ, as well as how they work and how much is known about their effects.

But people are also asking new questions. The growth of interest in a consumer view of health care has been at its strongest in birth control. Partly because of the growth of the women's movement, and its efforts to help women understand their own bodies and make their own decisions, birth control has come to be seen as the business primarily of the user, not the provider.

Users shop around not only between methods, but between places to get them. For example, the old division between those who went to clinics and those who went to their family practitioner has become more flexible. Those in search of contraception now go to either at different times, depending on convenience, the service they get and their perception of who is likely to be most helpful in meeting their particular needs.

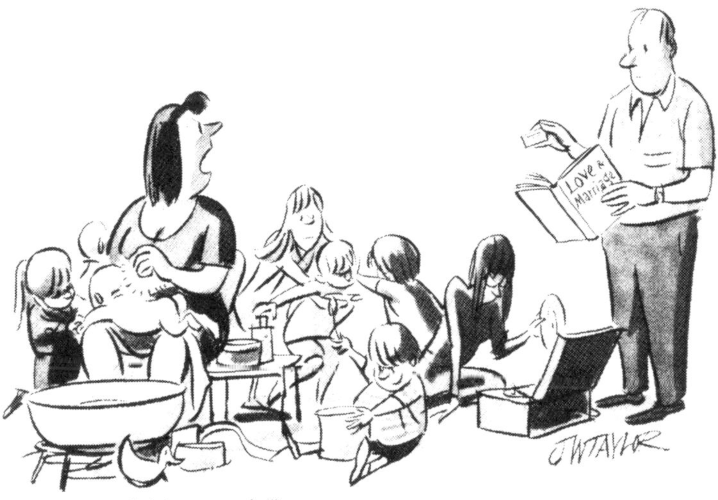

"Now you find the erratum slip!"

Providers of family planning services – administrators, medical staff, clinics and family practitioners – have begun to recognise that contraception has moved into the consumer age. So far, however, they have been better at seeing the need for change than at actually altering their approaches to meet consumer demand.

This latest version of the *Which?* Guide is an attempt to redress the balance. It is written for the consumer, from – we hope – the point of view of the consumer. It is less concerned with some medically fascinating but extremely rare side effect of a contraceptive than with the effects which may be felt by quite a number of people. It tries to bring out some of the practical snags and benefits of using different methods which may not normally be mentioned. It discusses the hurdles you may face in getting hold of, or getting the best service with, the different methods.

There is, unfortunately, no perfect method of birth control. There is not even a single 'best buy', and, given the time and phenomenal cost it takes to test a new contraceptive and put it on the market, it is unlikely that there will be in the foreseeable future. So we have approached the subject rather as we would the choice of cooker. Gas, or electricity? Do you normally cook for eight, or for two? Wall oven, or solid fuel centrepiece for a farmhouse kitchen? The choice depends on your lifestyle and needs (and constraints, like no gas laid on) rather than on any absolute standard.

It is just as feasible to make a sensible, informed choice on the right contraceptive for you. And if you make that choice, you are likely to find the contraceptive the most effective and trouble-free. There are a number of ways of measuring contraceptive efficiency (these are described in the Appendices) but we have given very little weight to these formal measures in describing the different types of contraceptive. This is because effectiveness in practice is linked with the user being happy with the method and so using it regularly. Only you can make that decision about which method it will be: nobody else should even try to.

Because we are more concerned with differences between methods than between brands, there is less 'product information' than there was in our first *Which?* Guide. Standards of quality control and of contraceptive testing have improved enormously since 1963, and there is no longer a need for us to look at different condoms, for instance, to see whether they will fail. The introduction of more methods involving doctors (Pills and coils) has meant there is far more monitoring and reporting on contraceptive side effects, as well as meaning that more methods are automatically subject to good quality control processes.

There is similarly less information than in the past on prices. This is partly because here again we are more concerned with methods than with brands, but partly because now that most contraceptives are free under the NHS, relative costs are less important to the consumer than to the doctor or administrator. So we have given an idea of cost only for the things you might buy for yourself.

Now that birth control has become standard practice for most people in Britain, and its users are beginning both to know and to ask more, there is no reason why an inadequate service should be acceptable. On the basis of a reasonable knowledge of what is available and possible, consumers should not only be able to make their own choices, but where those choices are restricted by the services available, should be able to articulate a demand for their improvement.

We may be stuck with the contraceptives around today but there is no reason why we should accept the services as they exist. If clinics in your area don't open at convenient times – for example, if there are no evening sessions – or have long waiting lists, or if you can't find their phone numbers in the directory or Yellow Pages (under Family Planning), complain to your Community Health Council or to the District Health Authority.

If your doctor is not particularly knowledgeable or helpful, go elsewhere – but preferably tell him, and even the Family Practitioner Committee, why you have decided to do so. A family doctor gets an item of service payment for attending to your contraceptive needs and that payment is just about as large as the one he gets for his overall care of you each year, so he ought to have a real financial incentive to do a good job. He also ought to have got himself properly trained, but unfortunately many have not undertaken the special training available, and rely on what they learnt at medical school and anything they have read since.

Better contraceptive – and abortion – services depend on well-informed consumers making those services into a consumer issue. If that happens, perhaps this really will be the last edition needed of our *Which?* Guide!

Controlling fertility: the points of intervention

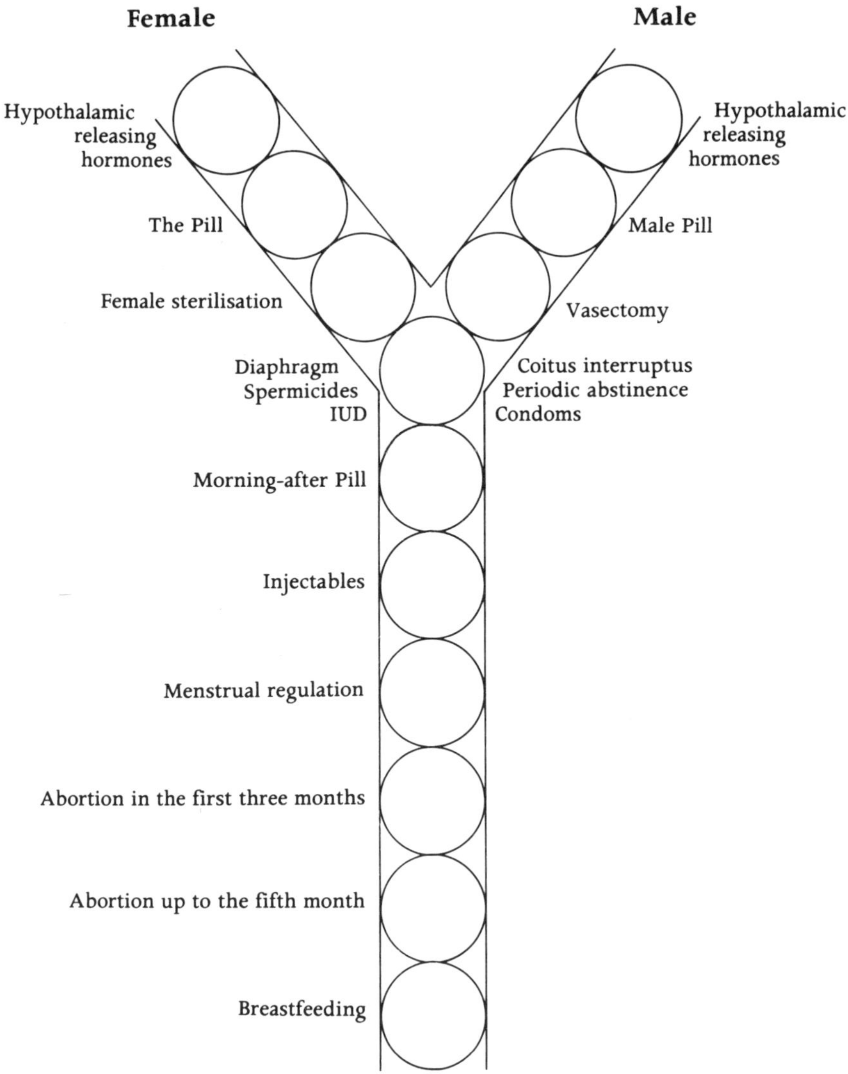

Controlling fertility

Contraception can be defined as an attempt to interfere with the normal process of reproduction. Because this process is quite a long one, in terms of time, and also quite a complicated one, there are all sorts of stages where you could in theory, or can in practice, intervene.

To illustrate this, we have used the idea of a Y, the left arm representing the woman's reproductive cycle and the right arm the man's, with the blobs at various points along each arm indicating what you can do to control your fertility, so that either sperm or egg is incapable of playing its part in the fertilisation process. At the junction of the Y are the methods which can be used to prevent sperm meeting egg. The tail of the Y shows the stages at which you can prevent a pregnancy developing after fertilisation has taken place.

A man's ability to father children depends on hormones produced at the base of the brain. The hypothalamus produces 'releasing' hormones which work on the pituitary which in turn produces two hormones which act on the testicles. These produce sperm, virtually continuously, in a complicated series of very small tubes in the testicles. Hundreds of millions are produced each day, and gradually mature as they move through these tubes and along the vas deferens. The vas deferens runs into the seminal vesicles, which produce and store most of the seminal fluid which in turn will provide nourishment and protection for the sperm. At orgasm, the semen – or seminal fluid, containing around 200 million sperm – shoots out along the urethra. The whole process takes approximately two to three months for a sperm to become fully mature and ready for ejaculation at orgasm.

It is extremely difficult to interfere with the production and development of sperm without affecting the male sex drive or the actual volume of semen secreted. Some of the efforts being made to do so are described in the chapter on New Horizons. The long time-lag between first production and ejaculation of the mature sperm leads to additional difficulties in designing a contraceptive to stop the process.

The next possibility of interference is to block the vas deferens along which the sperm has to pass. At the moment, this is done by cutting a small piece out of the vas, and sealing the ends that remain: vasectomy. In theory, it should be possible to block the tubes in a less drastic way, so that the passage of sperm can be restored when required, but so far attempts have resulted either in a less than effective blockage, or in a build-up of fibrous tissue around the damaged area of vas, which makes it difficult for sperm to get through even after the tube has been rejoined or the block removed.

The simplest way of intervening in male fertility is to stop the semen, when it appears at the time of ejaculation, from reaching the woman's egg. This can be achieved in a number of ways. Periodic abstinence – having sex only at those times in the woman's cycle when there is no egg ready for fertilisation; coitus interruptus – when the man withdraws from the vagina immediately before he ejaculates; and the use of condoms, diaphragms and spermicides to prevent semen reaching the vagina; are all comparatively simple contraceptive techniques with a long history.

The reproductive process in women may seem rather more complicated than the production, development and ejaculation of sperm is in the man, but in some ways it offers greater opportunities for contraceptive intervention.

The control centre of the woman's menstrual cycle is also the hypothalamus in the brain. This sends information by means of releasing hormones to the pituitary gland, which produces two hormones called the follicle-stimulating hormone (FSH) and luteinising hormone (LH). These act on the ovum, or egg, to ripen the egg cell and prepare for conception. The hormones also control the level of the steroids oestrogen and progesterone in the blood.

Each woman is born with a lifetime's supply of eggs which are stored in the ovary, and never produces more. Generally, one is ripened every month and FSH, which is more active during the first half of the cycle, plays a large

The male reproductive system

Side view

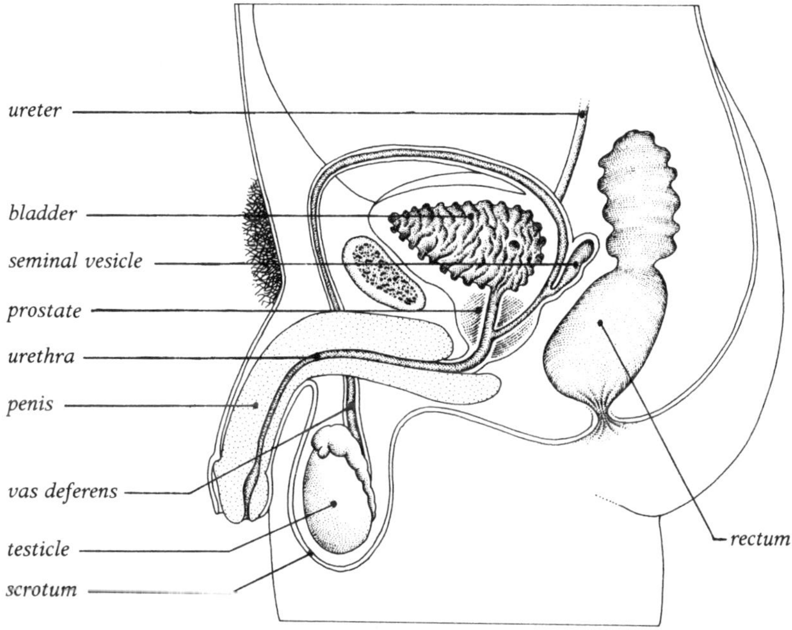

Front view

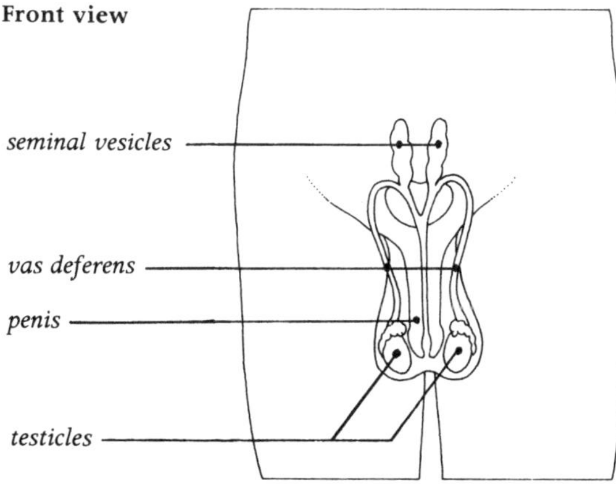

Male methods

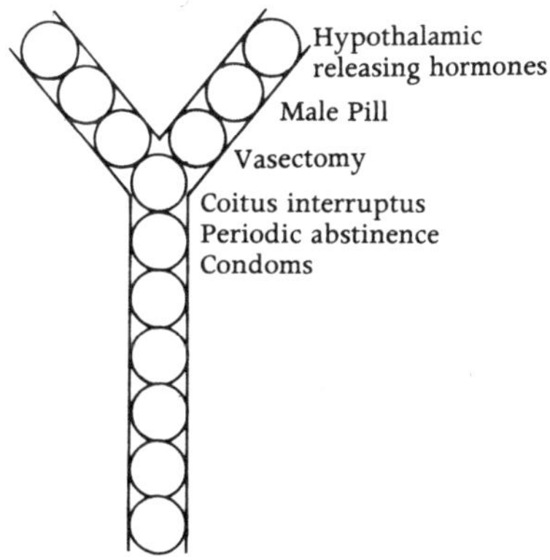

part in its ripening. The ripening ovarian follicle, or egg case, produces oestrogen at ovulation. The follicle ruptures and the ripened egg is released from the ovary to pass down the Fallopian tube.

When the egg is released, the ovarian hormones oestrogen and progesterone act on the lining of the womb to prepare it for the implantation of a fertilised egg. The lining becomes thicker, with more blood going through it.

If the egg is not fertilised, or if a fertilised egg is not implanted in the lining of the womb, the oestrogen and progesterone levels in the body begin to fall again, the lining of the womb comes away and is shed, and menstrual bleeding begins, lasting from three to seven days. When the oestrogen levels fall, the pituitary gland releases FSH and the whole cycle begins again.

Because the release of hormones from the pituitary gland in the woman follows a predictable cycle, it is comparatively simple to produce artificial steroids which suppress the production and release of those hormones at the pituitary level. When this is done, no egg ripens and the menstrual cycle described is prevented from being triggered off. The artificial steroids, oestrogen and progestagen, are given in the form of the Pill or by an injection; various other ways of getting them into the body are being tested.

If an egg is released from the ovary, however, the next possible point of intervention is to interrupt its journey down the Fallopian tube. Like vasectomy for the man, this is done by means of a simple operation in which the tube is cut or blocked. While the vas deferens in men is very near the surface of the scrotum and is therefore easy to get at, the Fallopian tubes are tucked away inside the woman's body and are more difficult to reach. Modern sterilisation techniques have been developed to cope with this difficulty.

If a fertilised egg does reach the womb, it is also possible to stop it becoming embedded in the womb's lining.

During the three or four days the egg takes to travel along the Fallopian tubes, become fertilised and reach the womb,

The female reproductive system

Side view

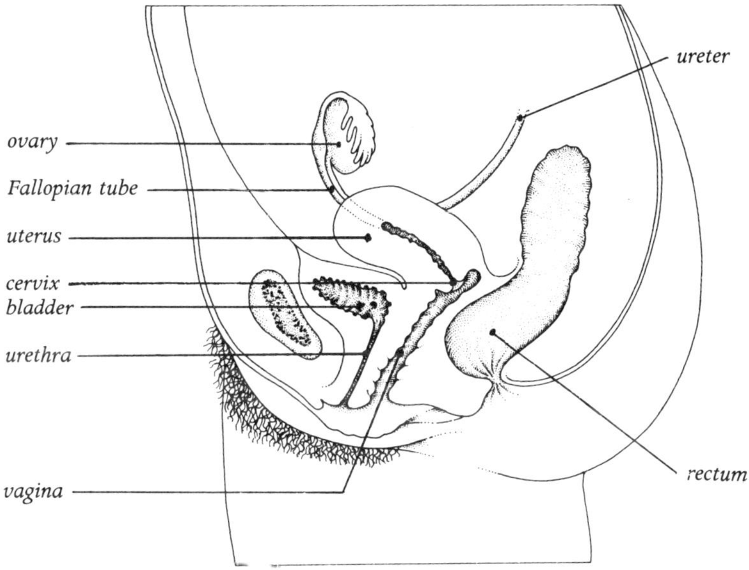

Front view

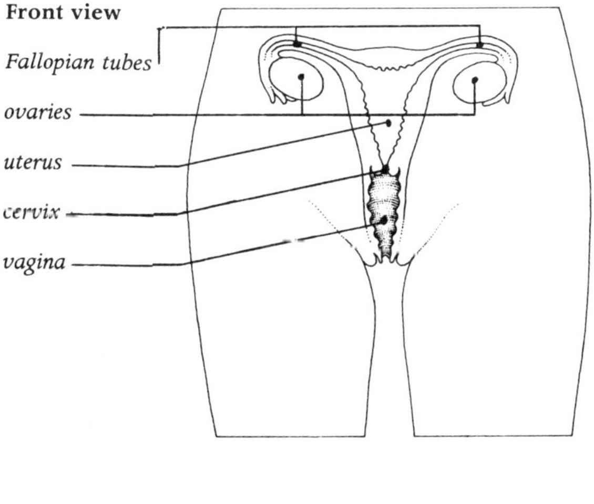

Female methods

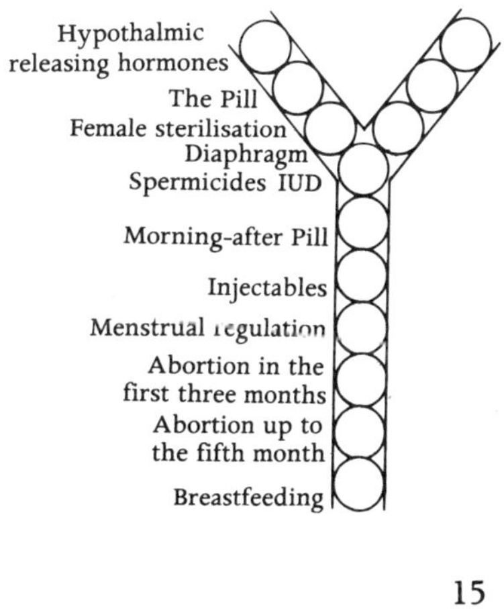

it is possible to create an environment in the womb which is somehow unfavourable both to the egg and to the sperm, which are at a very delicate stage in their development. Some oral contraceptives, and the IUD, are believed to work in that way.

Once a fertilised egg has been implanted and has begun to grow in the womb, it can only be removed along with the womb's lining. A substance called prostaglandin can be used to make the womb contract and bring on a period. Alternatively, a narrow cannula (a surgical tube) can be inserted through the cervix into the womb and its contents taken out by suction. Or, if the pregnancy has developed further, a standard abortion may be carried out.

Each of the different points at which you can intervene to control fertility has different advantages and disadvantages. The earlier in the male or female reproductive cycle the intervention is, the more remote it is from the sex act or pregnancy. The remoteness from sex can help to make it a more reliable intervention, too – the user doesn't have to think of contraception at a time when his or her mind would rather be on other things. On the other hand, the further away from the act of sex the intervention is, the more likely it is to involve substances like hormones, which have widespread effects not just on the reproductive system, but on the whole body.

In the later stages of the reproductive cycle, after the sex act and when conception may have occurred, you are moving towards moral questions (over when life begins and what you define as an abortion) and legal problems.

Where the three strokes of the Y join, you have the methods which, with the exception of the IUD, are directly connected with the sex act, have fewer ill effects, but are more tedious to use and have a higher failure rate.

Most people choose different contraceptives and abortifacients from along the spectrum at different times in their lives, depending on what fits best with their lives at any particular point.

Traditional methods

Contraception isn't new: people have been trying for thousands of years to control the size and the timing of their families. In Britain, as in many other countries, the most widely used methods were probably breastfeeding, coitus interruptus or 'withdrawal', a variety of home-made tampons or pessaries, and abortion – backed up with some discreet infanticide. The interest in a more 'natural' way of life has revived interest in some of these techniques.

Breastfeeding

When you are pregnant, your body contains high levels of both oestrogen and progesterone, as well as another steroid called prolactin, which is involved in breast-milk production. After the baby is born, the levels of oestrogen and progesterone fall and you begin to produce breast-milk. It is thought that the high level of oestrogen actually prevents the milk being produced – this is why if you start to use a Pill which contains both oestrogen and progestagen (the combined Pill) when you are breastfeeding, it will reduce the amount of milk and the time that it lasts.

While prolactin is present in the system, you produce much less of the luteinising hormone LH which acts as a trigger for your reproductive cycle. Exactly how these two hormones work together, and on the other hormones involved, is not clear, but the overall effect is that even if you have some irregular bleeding during this time, you are unlikely to be having a proper menstrual cycle, leading to a ripe egg being released into the womb.

Background

Breastfeeding has had an effect on the number of children people have throughout the world, but surprisingly little good information exists about how it works and how effective it is for the individual woman. This is because the hormonal changes associated with breastfeeding are quite a complicated subject and researchers are not always asking the same questions. For instance, in many countries it used to be the rule that if you were breastfeeding you did not have sex. Obviously, you didn't get pregnant either – but that did not prove that breastfeeding kept you temporarily infertile. And breastfeeding itself is a word that covers all sorts of different practices – is the baby getting supplementary foods? is it fed 'on demand' or only at certain intervals?

So all that can really be said is that if you take a group of women who are not using any contraceptive, there will on average be a longer gap between babies if they are breastfeeding than if they are not, and that the longer they are breastfeeding, the longer that gap tends to be – but only slightly. People like demographers, who are looking at whole populations, can therefore say that breastfeeding has an effect on the overall fertility of that population. When it comes to any particular woman, though, there is so much variation that she would be unwise to rely on breastfeeding to stop herself getting pregnant.

Safety

There are much better reasons for breastfeeding than any contraceptive effect it may have. Breast-milk helps to protect a baby from various infections, as well as being designed by nature to be the best possible mix of nutrients for it – at least for the first four or five months. After that the milk has to be supplemented, and so any contraceptive value of breastfeeding will be lessened.

Effectiveness

As we have already said, this is not a reliable method of contraception. If you are breastfeeding there is likely to be a longer time before you begin to menstruate, but somewhere between 3 and 7 per cent of women actually get pregnant again before menstruating, so you cannot assume that you will continue to be infertile until you start to menstruate normally again.

If you are breastfeeding, and don't want to start another baby straight away, you should supplement any contraceptive effect breastfeeding has with another method, such as the progestagen-only Pill, an IUD, spermicides or other barrier methods, or an injectable – none of which affects the quantity or quality of breast-milk.

'Withdrawal' or coitus interruptus

This is one of the world's oldest real contraceptive methods, which is often called 'being careful'. The size of families fell in Britain a hundred years ago, before any of the 'modern' methods were available except for the condom, mainly because of 'withdrawal'.

It works by the man withdrawing his penis just before ejaculation, so that the sperm do not get into the vagina and therefore cannot travel up to meet the egg.

Background

In Britain withdrawal is still the third most popular method, after condoms and the Pill. Family planning experts used rather to frown on it, probably because satisfied users never bothered to go to a clinic, so the only ones they came across were those who were not happy with the method and wanted an alternative. Additionally, early family planners were often feminists, who doubted the willingness or reliability of many men in using the method. As a consequence of the experts' lack of interest, there are very few studies of the method, its efficiency or why people use it.

Safety and effectiveness

The very few studies on failure rates suggest that coitus interruptus is generally a moderately reliable method, which can be more effective among users who are happy with it and carry it out dependably. Most of the failures probably come about as a result of the man not withdrawing his penis quickly enough.

It is often said that there are failures with this method because even before ejaculation a little fluid tends to dribble from the penis, and may contain a few sperm. But as more research is done into couples who are sub-fertile, it has begun to be accepted that there may have to be an awful lot of sperm around before there is any likelihood that one will manage to fertilise an egg, and that is why a normal ejaculation contains hundreds of millions of sperm. If this is so, it is very unlikely that you would get pregnant from the odd sperm which may be leaked before ejaculation.

It also used to be said that withdrawal could have psychological consequences, and that the abrupt end to sex led to tension and frustration. While the abrupt ending may be a factor in how acceptable you find the method, there is no evidence that it causes any psychological damage.

Acceptability

Some couples are sufficiently happy with coitus interruptus – no side effects, nothing to buy or have to talk to others about, easy to use – to rely on it as a routine method of contraception. Many more use it as an occasional method, or as a back-up method to something else, such as periodic abstinence.

For people having casual sex it has the advantage of not needing advance planning, or the continuing use of a contraceptive with side effects. Against that, the woman may not be confident that a casual partner will be sufficiently careful in withdrawing, and as she is probably very unwilling to become pregnant, its failure rate may be too high for her.

It is a useful emergency method if you have forgotten to take the Pill or have run out of spermicides, or left the cap behind, and so on. It is also a very good combination method if you don't want to use one of the most reliable ones, like the combined Pill or IUD, but do want a higher level of efficiency than you will get with periodic abstinence alone. (A very large proportion of people do in fact use more than one method of contraception at a time.)

Because of the absence of side effects or of any mechanical interference with the act of sex, couples may use it happily for years. Whether you would choose it as a permanent method depends partly on how much you mind the possibility of a pregnancy, or the abrupt end to the sex act itself, as well as how easy you and your partner find it to practice. Although it is usually described as one of the few male methods around, it really needs the cooperation of both partners, which can be a bonus for those who believe that contraception should be a joint affair. Certainly it is a discreet method, and one which is simply a private matter between the two people concerned.

Home-made tampons and pessaries

These, which have been described all over the world, are vaginal plugs designed to stop the sperm getting up into the womb. They can be made of almost anything – rags, sponges, dung, for instance – and are often used together with something designed to be a kind of spermicide, like vinegar, sea-water or an acid plant-juice. We don't recommend that you use any of these, but anyone interested in home-made tampons and pessaries should read on.

You can make a vaginal barrier from a 15 cm square piece of cloth (it should be clean and soft) folded with the frayed edges inside and sewn together with thread. You should leave a free end of thread to help in removing the pad. Clean cotton or silk waste can be cut and rolled into a tampon about the size of a hen's egg, and held together with a thread which should have a long end for removal. Another alternative is a small sponge, either a sea sponge or a foam rubber one, cut to size and enclosed in a fine net with a thread attached. Ordinary small commercial menstrual tampons can also be used.

Any of these barriers should be soaked or smeared with a spermicide. This can either be a commercially available spermicide (which will be more effective) or a home-made preparation of vinegar or lemon juice mixed with boiled water – one part vinegar or lemon to 20 parts water. You could use a cubic cm of mild soap dissolved in a litre of boiled water, or any edible oil or fat. (Never use strong soap, soap powder or detergents, mustard oil or a strong salt solution: they will irritate or even injure your vagina.)

Background

Sponges and similar barriers were popular with the early family planners, when there was not much around in the way of other methods, because they were cheap and easy to make at home. Like so many other 'natural' methods they are now having something of a revival, though again like so many of the barrier methods there has been almost no work on them to see how effective, acceptable and safe they are.

Quite a lot of work is now being done to develop new, improved, vaginal barriers and these are described under New Horizons. The ones described here are the traditional varieties, which may be useful in an emergency.

Safety and Effectiveness

None of these vaginal barriers will do you any harm, provided they are clean and you take care what you use as a spermicide. It is probable that they are less effective than a diaphragm or cap used with a commercial spermicide, but they are quite untested.

The barrier should be left in place for at least six hours after the last act of intercourse, and should be washed in mild soapy water, rinsed and dried before using again.

Acceptability

If you favour self-sufficiency and the natural life, these barrier methods may be an attractive proposition, assuming that you are not worried by a comparatively high chance of pregnancy. Otherwise, you would probably feel that a diaphragm and commercial spermicide require less effort, even if they do necessitate a fitting at a clinic or doctor's. The drawbacks are basically the same as for other barrier methods: they are awkward to carry around with you and need to be inserted just before the act of sex. With a commercial spermicide, or some of the home-made ones, you may find the extra slipperiness of the vagina decreases sensation (or improves it, if you tend to be dry). On the other hand, some of the barriers can be so absorbent that you may find your vagina very dry, making sex uncomfortable. These natural vaginal barriers have a distinct advantage as an emergency method, because they are made out of things which you will normally have around the house.

Douching

Douching – washing out the vagina after sex to get rid of the sperm – has also been used for a long time by people trying to avoid getting pregnant. You can buy a douching syringe at a chemist's.

Unfortunately, although water does have a spermicidal effect, douching does not work as a contraceptive. When you have sex, the sperm swim into the cervix within seconds of ejaculation. By the time you have been able to use a douche, they are already likely to be way beyond the vagina, which is the only part the douche will wash, and any remaining sperm around the cervix are just as likely to be helped on their way by the douche as washed away.

If, for personal reasons, you like to douche, that is up to you – though it is unnecessary for hygiene. You should never douche after sex if you have been using a spermicide, as you will lessen its effect (see the Spermicides section). Don't think of douching as a contraceptive – it isn't.

Barrier methods

Condoms

Condoms are sheaths of latex rubber designed to cover the erect penis and contain the semen which is ejaculated. They are around seven inches long (but will fit closely to most sizes and shapes of penis) and generally have a teat at the end to leave space for the semen.

Background

Currently used by some two million people in Britain, they are one of the best-known and longest established contraceptives. Earlier forms of condom, made of skin or animal gut, were popular in the seventeenth century as a prevention against venereal disease, and in the nineteenth century they were, with coitus interruptus, probably the main reason for declining birth rates in Britain (the head of Queen Victoria was stamped on one brand!)

Their long history probably explains the variety of names they go by – sheath, rubber, protective, prophylactic and preventative, as well as French letter (the French return the compliment with 'capote anglaise'). Many of the names indicate their use against sexually transmitted diseases; this may help to explain the improper – or even slightly squalid – aura associated with them, which later carried over to other contraceptive methods as they were developed.

Modern condoms are generally lubricated, which makes them easier to put on (they are gently unrolled over the erect penis) and easier, once on, to insert into the vagina. It is claimed that lubrication also helps to make up for the loss of sensitivity for both partners. They come in a variety of colours and some have bumps or ridges on them which are supposed to increase the woman's enjoyment, though some women dislike them and others don't notice the difference. There is even a narrower brand for those men who have a smaller penis.

The majority of condoms used in this country are made by London Rubber Company Products Limited, although there are quite a number of small manufacturers or importers. London Rubber sell under the brand name Durex as

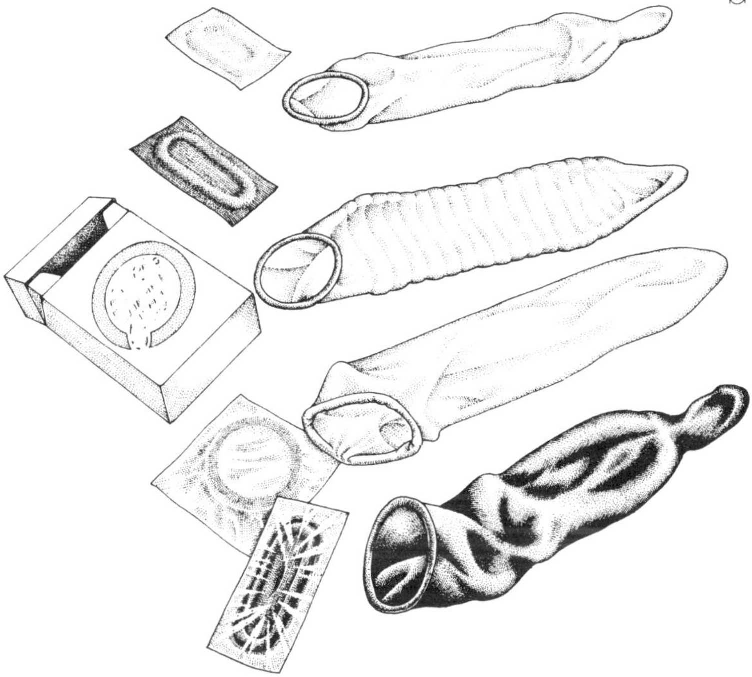

well as under various other brand names, and they additionally manufacture for a number of mail order firms who sell them under their own brand names. Family Planning Sales Limited, which covenants its profits to the Family Planning Association, also has two brand-name condoms (one, Two's Company, is a pack also containing spermicides) which they sell by mail order and through a few other outlets, as well as to clinics.

Safety

A very few people may be allergic to one or more ingredients in a rubber condom, and develop a skin irritation. Others may be allergic to the lubricant, if the condom is a lubricated brand, or to the spermicide, if the condom is one which has a spermicide with the lubricant. Either partner, of course, could develop the irritation. London Rubber make a condom called Durex Allergy, designed to help if you suffer from an allergy to the usual lubricant. If that does not work, it may be worth trying other brands to see if you can identify what is causing the problem – even if it turns out to be the ingredients in the rubber, different condoms have a slightly different mix of ingredients and you may find one which suits you. Unfortunately, the process of trial and error can be very uncomfortable, for those very few people who suffer from an allergy; you may simply decide to switch to another method without more ado.

Otherwise there are no ill-effects associated with condoms. If one slips off inside the vagina it cannot get 'lost' and is easily retrievable using a finger.

It has long been recognised that condoms help to prevent the spread of sexually transmitted diseases (though if you have the slightest reason to think you have or your partner might have a sexually transmitted disease, don't rely on a condom – go to a special clinic, or see your family practitioner, and get it diagnosed and treated.)

There is a little evidence, but not very conclusive, that condoms may also help to reduce cervical cancer. Cervical cancer is associated, among other things, with the age at which the woman first had sex and the number of sexual partners she has had; it is also now thought to be associated with the number of partners the man has had. (Studies of cervical cancer tend to look either at any differences between Pill- and IUD-users in the numbers developing cancer, or at differences between users, of both Pill and IUD, and non-users.)

Because condoms (like diaphragms) have been regarded as a 'non-medical' method, very little research has been done into medical conditions which may or may not be associated with them. This means that there is little proof that condoms have any beneficial effect – or indeed that they are harmful, though given their very widespread use over time it is probable that any very serious ill-effect would have been noticed by now, if only accidentally.

Effectiveness

Good condoms, used regularly, may have a failure rate as low as two per hundred user-years. Generally, the failure rate is higher. One reason could be poor-quality condoms. Not all those sold in Britain conform to British Standard BS 3704 (you can tell which do because they carry the 'kite-mark'), although all manufacturers carry out their own tests. There is as yet no single internationally recognised standard for condom testing, so you cannot assume that the ones which don't carry the kite-mark are as reliable as those that do. We recommend you stick to kite-marked brands.

One perennial old wives' tale associated with condoms is that the manufacturers must by law puncture a certain number to appease the susceptibility of various religious groups. This is not true.

Some brands of condom are advertised as being spermicidal – the lubricant on them contains a spermicide. While this may provide some extra protection, it is unlikely to be quite as effective as a traditional spermicide used together with an ordinary condom, and if you want to maximise reliability we recommend you use a separate spermicide (see the section on Spermicides).

However good they are when they leave the manufacturers, condoms can deteriorate over time or if they are badly stored. There is a 'use before . . .' date on brands conforming to British Standards, but like the date-stamp on foods, it is a guideline rather than a guarantee. If rubber is kept in a warm damp atmosphere it may deteriorate. If a condom is kept for a long time in a wallet or similar container, the sealed pack may wear and cease to be airtight, and again the condom will deteriorate. Condoms should be looked after carefully and used as soon as possible after being bought.

They are also less effective if they are not properly used. Condoms are made of extremely thin rubber and may tear if they catch on a ring or a fingernail when being put on, so they need to be handled carefully. The tip of the condom

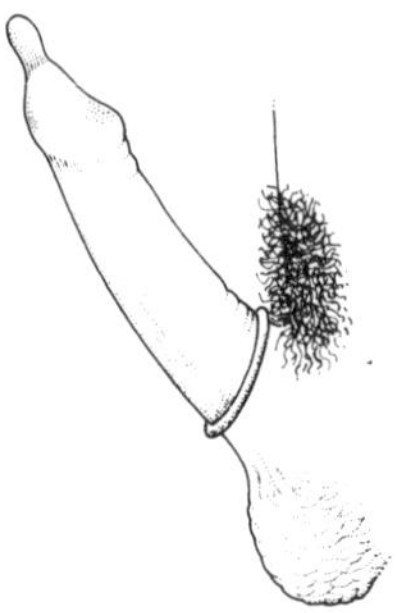

should be squeezed as it is rolled on to leave the end empty of air. Less strain is then put on the condom and it is less likely to burst or leak. Some couples find that smearing a little spermicidal jelly or lubricating cream on the condom once it has been put on, helps it to slide into the vagina more easily, and minimises the danger of it tearing.

A condom should be put on before intercourse. If you rely on withdrawing and putting it on immediately before orgasm, you may be too late.

After orgasm, you should withdraw your penis before the erection has subsided, holding the condom on the penis as you do so – otherwise it may slip off and be left in the vagina, or the semen may run out into the vagina.

Acceptability

Condoms have often been recommended above all for occasional use, or casual sexual encounters. They can certainly be a very useful method in such circumstances (and their value in protecting against sexually transmitted diseases may be a bonus in casual encounters) because they are easily available, unobtrusive to carry with you, and do not require advance planning for use. However, some people – perhaps particularly young people – find the last-moment fumbling while attempting to disguise what is happening very awkward. Unless you feel that you can carry off the situation comfortably, another method may be preferable.

Between couples who know each other well the situation may be different. Either partner may put on the condom, making the action a part of the love-play. Condoms may be the preferred method for long-term use, or they may be used for emergencies – for example, in the rest of the cycle if the woman has missed her Pill for two or three days, or if her IUD has fallen out, or if she is between methods, or has just had a baby.

Even the best condom will dull sensation a little for the man. This can be an advantage if he tends to reach orgasm too quickly, but others may find it reduces their enjoyment of sex substantially. Some women, too, can feel the difference a condom makes and it may affect their pleasure. The need to remove the condom before the penis becomes limp can mean that the act of sex finishes rather quickly, which may be upsetting for some couples.

Disposing of condoms occasionally causes difficulty or embarrassment. If the open end is twisted around itself and tied, a condom can be flushed down a lavatory – if left open, it will tend to float. But with the end tied, they are a real nuisance for sewage-workers, so you have to choose between your care for the environment and your possible embarrassment, and it would be best to find some other method of disposal.

Availability

Condoms are fairly widely available from a variety of sources. Traditionally, the barber was a provider of condoms and, if you can still find a barber, he probably still is. Chemists, another traditional source, have become slightly less embarrassing to visit since most of them now carry condoms displayed on their counters, so the buyer does not necessarily have to ask for them but merely picks them up and presents them for payment. However, young people particularly may still find the confrontation awkward.

This probably explains the popularity of mail order and of condom-vending machines. Mail order condom supplies are widely advertised in local newspapers and magazines, and if you are not keen on the plain brown envelope arriving at your home you may well find that somebody where you work buys bulk supplies on mail order and retails them to his or her fellow-workers. Vending machines, though discreet and useful, have a poor reputation: it is said that many are left empty deliberately (especially in pubs) on the well-founded assumption that many people will be too shy in a crowded bar to go and demand their money back if the machine has swallowed their coins but not produced a packet of condoms.

The only place you cannot get condoms from is your family practitioner via the National Health Service. All other methods are freely available on the NHS, but when family planning became part of it in 1974 no arrangements were made for GPs to offer condom prescriptions. If you decide to switch from one brand of Pill to another, your GP can prescribe both and will probably tell you to use an additional method for the first two weeks on the second Pill – but he cannot prescribe that method if it is a condom. So you will have to pay unless you go to a family planning clinic (these come under a different part of the NHS) where you can get regular supplies of condoms free of charge.

The average price for a packet of three lubricated condoms is about 50 pence. Large chains of chemists usually offer a discount below the recommended retail price, and mail order firms offer bulk savings.

Summary

Condoms are pretty reliable and virtually free of side effects. If you don't need contraception all the time they may be an excellent choice so long as you are not worried about getting hold of them, or of the mechanics of using them. They are a very good back-up or emergency method for couples temporarily in need of an alternative method, and for those who want a regular method which is free of possible long-term ill effects. As one of the only three male methods widely available, they may particularly appeal to those who believe men should play a greater part in contraception.

They may be less attractive to those who like to keep contraception well apart from the spontaneity of sex; to those who consider that the onus is on the woman to prevent herself getting pregnant; to the shy; and to those who find that condoms noticeably diminish sexual pleasure.

Diaphragms

Diaphragms are shallow domes of rubber with a metal rim. The rim – which is also encased in rubber – may be a flat compressible band (the 'flat spring' diaphragm) or a wire

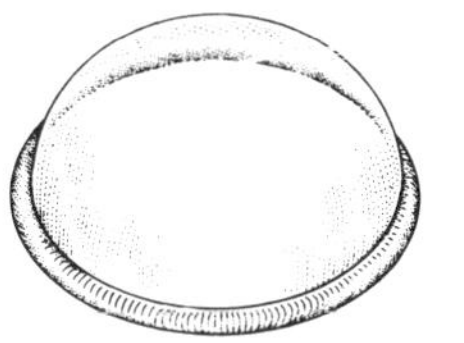

spiral (the 'coil spring' diaphragm). They are designed to fit over the cervix and work both by acting as a barrier to prevent the sperm reaching the womb, and by being a receptacle to hold spermicide near the cervix. As diaphragms, however well fitted, do not sit tightly enough against the cervix to prevent completely the live sperm getting past, the second function – keeping the spermicide in place – is probably the more important one.

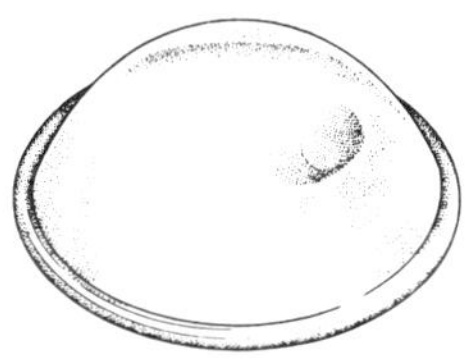

Background

Early versions of diaphragms are known from many parts of the world. Discs of oiled silk paper were used in China and Japan; moulded wax wafers and even moulded opium cups have been described in Europe and the Far East. The hollowed-out skin of half a fruit, such as a lemon, was another widely used alternative.

The modern diaphragm was invented in 1838, following the discovery of vulcanised rubber, but only drew widespread attention in the 1880s. It is often called a 'Dutch cap', a tribute to a Dutchman who was an early promoter of the method. It became popular with the early family planners, many of whom were feminists, because it offered women a method they could use and control, but during the 1960s and 1970s it lost ground rapidly as the Pill and the IUD were introduced. Today it is making a limited come-back, especially in some feminist groups and among women concerned with the long-term effects of Pill or IUD use.

There are two brands approved by the FPA; a flat spring diaphragm under the Durex brand name made by LRC, and a coil spring model made by Ortho Pharmaceuticals Limited.

Safety

A very few women may be unable to use a diaphragm or one of the caps because their vagina is long or their cervix is too short, so that they either cannot reach the cervix easily or cannot ensure that the diaphragm or cap is properly placed. A few others may have damaged the cervix or the vaginal muscles during childbirth or there may be a prolapse. The person doing the fitting should be able to tell this and advise on possible alternatives. There should be something to suit most women – see particularly the section on Caps.

A very few people may be allergic to one or more ingredients in the rubber of a diaphragm, but this seems to be less of a problem than it is with condoms. (There may be problems with spermicides – see that section.)

Diaphragms, like condoms, have not been studied very much and there is little medical literature about any possible ill-effects. However, given their steady use over almost a century, it is probable that any serious ill-effects would have been noticed. One ill-effect which has been found among diaphragm-users is a greater tendency to cystitis, and other minor problems associated with the urinary tract.

There is a little evidence, but not very conclusive, that the use of diaphragms with spermicides may help to limit the spread of sexually transmitted diseases and other vaginal infections. If this is so, it seems to be an effect of the spermicide , rather than of the diaphragm itself, and is discussed under the spermicide section.

There is also some evidence that rates of cervical cancer are lower among diaphragm-users than among users of the Pill and the IUD. Because there are many factors which seem to increase or decrease the risk of cervical cancer, including the age of first sexual experience, the number of partners, and so on, it has not been possible to compare diaphragm-users with other women on all those possible risk factors. So it is not clear whether it is the diaphragm which has a protective effect, or whether women who choose a diaphragm are of a particular type.

Effectiveness

Used regularly and carefully, the diaphragm and spermicide together may have a failure rate as low as two per hundred user-years. Generally, the failure rate is higher. This may be due to the deterioration of the diaphragm over time or because it is badly stored or just through use. If rubber is kept in a warm damp atmosphere it will deteriorate. After use, a diaphragm must be carefully washed in ordinary soap and water, rinsed out thoroughly, and dried before being stored in its container. It can be powdered with starch after being dried but this is not necessary. It should never be powdered with talc: this used to be recommended but it has been found that the talc itself can have harmful effects if absorbed into the vagina.

Diaphragms may lose their effectiveness if over time the rim becomes bent out of its circular shape, or if the cap is stretched so that the rubber weakens. They are quite strong but will not survive snags from fingernails or rings. Properly treated one should last at least a year. It should be examined at intervals, being held up to a strong light to look for thin patches, holes or cracks, especially where the rim joins the dome.

A diaphragm can be put in at any time before sex, depending on what is convenient. Before putting it in, two strips about 2.5 cm long should be squeezed from the tube of spermicide on to each side of the diaphragm, then smeared over the surface and round the rim. However, if the time gap between putting it in and having sex is more than two hours, most of the spermicide will have seeped away and an additional spermicidal cream or suppository should be put in the vagina.

To put in a diaphragm, squeeze it into a long oval and then slide it into the vagina as far as it will go, until the back end slides beyond the cervix. The front end can then be pushed up to lie behind the pubic bone. The rim regains its regular shape when you let go of it, and presses against the walls of the vagina on all sides. It stays in place partly by the tension of the rim and partly because of the vaginal muscles. The dome can be either upwards or downwards, depending on individual taste – whichever way is the more comfortable.

The woman will need to check that the diaphragm is in

Inserting a diaphragm or cap

You can insert the diaphragm or cap in the position you find the most comfortable

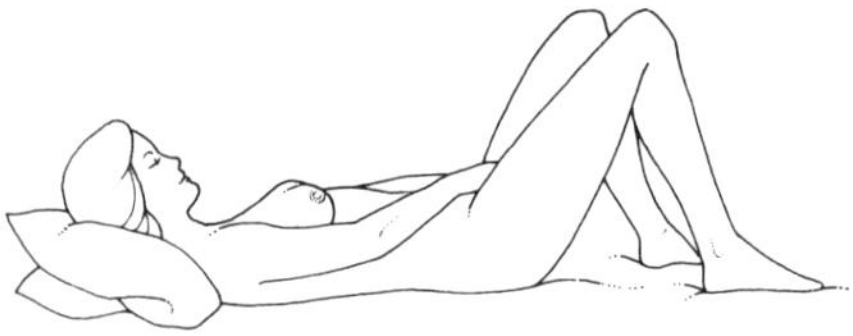

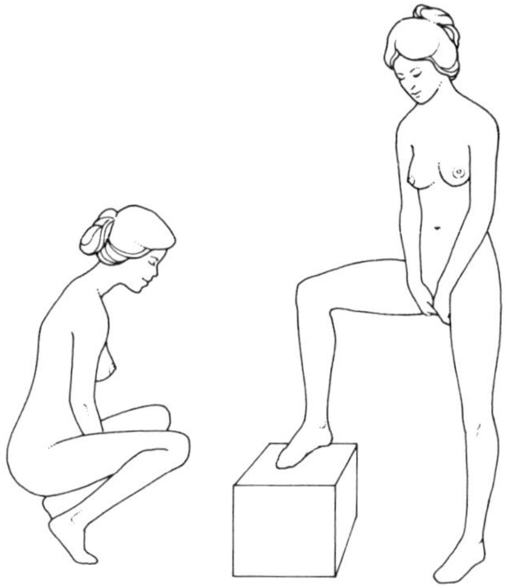

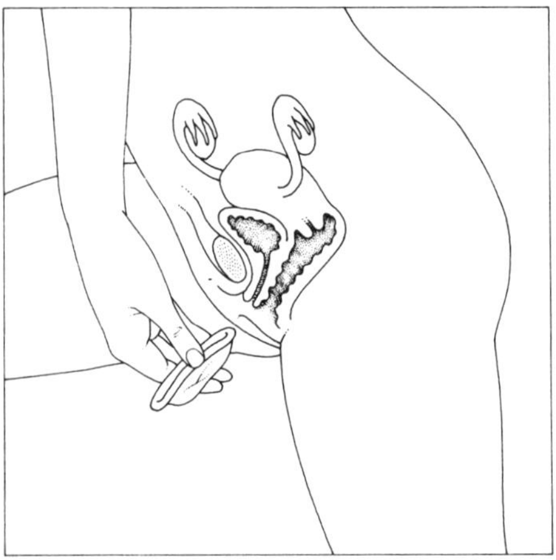

To put in a diaphragm, squeeze it into a long oval and then slide it into the vagina as far as it will go, until the back end slides beyond the cervix

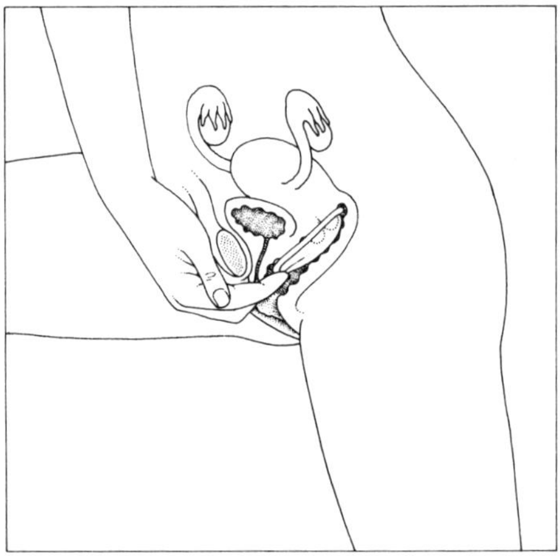

The front end can then be pushed up to lie behind the pubic bone

correctly – it should be possible to feel the cervix as a hard protuberance through the thin rubber. Occasionally by mistake the diaphragm may be put in with its back edge in front of the cervix, in which case, on checking, the cervix can be felt directly, uncovered.

After intercourse the diaphragm should be left in place for at least six hours. If the couple have sex more than once during that time, the diaphragm should *not* be taken out. Instead, additional spermicide should be put into the vagina each time, and the diaphragm should be left in place for at least six hours after the last act.

The diaphragm is unlikely to be dislodged while it is left in the vagina. Urinating will not disturb it, but during a bowel movement the cap may be dislodged by straining and should be held in place by one finger. This is not very likely to happen with a diaphragm – it is more common with a vault or cervical cap – so if it does it may be an indication that the size needs checking.

It does not matter if a period starts while the diaphragm is in place. Blood will get past it, so leave it in if that is more convenient. Incidentally, during a period intercourse may be more pleasant if there is a diaphragm in place because it does hold back some of the flow.

Another point which could affect the reliability of the diaphragm is that the size of the vagina may change. If a woman fitted for a diaphragm has not previously had sexual intercourse she should go back for a refit after the first six weeks. After any vaginal operation, after having a baby, during the menopause or if there is any substantial gain or loss – say 10 lbs (or 4½ kilos) – in weight, she should also have the diaphragm fitting checked. In any case the fitting should be checked once a year.

Acceptability

Women who dislike touching their vulva, or have cultural taboos about it, will find using a diaphragm inappropriate. Some people are uneasy about the premeditated aspect –

'going to a party with your diaphragm in' – and may prefer a method like the Pill or the IUD which is so remote from the act of sex that they can largely forget about it.

For some, the presence of a spermicide is an advantage, because it helps to lubricate the vagina; others – both men and women – find the spermicide too slippery, affecting the amount of sensation they experience. While many people do not notice the diaphragm during the act of sex, others – again, both men and women – may feel it quite noticeably and even experience discomfort, especially if the penis hits the rim. Different sexual positions may make it more or less noticeable. If a diaphragm suddenly begins to be painful during intercourse, it is an indication that a different one may be needed.

Some women like to wash after intercourse, particularly when using a spermicide which tends to leak a little. Washing is fine, but douching cannot be done if a diaphragm is used: it removes the protection needed to make sure the sperm are no longer active and it may even wash some active sperm up into the cervical canal.

The diaphragm is bulky to carry, especially when the supply of spermicide is added, which may be a disadvantage if the woman is away from home. It may also be difficult to conceal from other members of the family or those with whom she lives.

Like condoms, diaphragms – indeed, all caps – are instantly effective, which makes them a very useful method for those who have sex only occasionally and so do not wish to use a more permanent method of contraception. They are also an excellent fall-back method if a couple of Pills have been missed, or if the woman is about to have an IUD fitted, or is waiting for her partner's vasectomy to reveal a clear sperm count, for example.

They are probably less satisfactory for use in casual sexual encounters, or for those who find the mechanics of contraception embarrassing.

Women who are unhappy about possible ill-effects of the

Pill and IUD, and who like a method which is very much in their own hands and under their control, and who are interested in and at ease with their own bodies, often find a diaphragm an extremely good method of contraception.

Availability

Diaphragms need to be fitted by properly trained people (though not necessarily medically qualified ones). In Britain, they are generally fitted by a doctor or nurse, and therefore a woman who wants one will have to go to her family practitioner or family planning clinic. Some GPs are enthusiastic about diaphragms and those over 40 may be the most experienced in fitting them – indeed it is often said that a high proportion of older doctors' wives use them. Other GPs are less interested and may be unwilling to undertake the fitting. If your own doctor is unwilling to prescribe this particular form of contraception you may go for contraceptive services to another doctor within the area run by your Family Practitioner Committee. A list of doctors in the area willing to see contraceptive clients from other GPs' lists should be available from post offices, as well as from the Family Practitioner Committee. However, this list does not distinguish between the methods doctors are willing to prescribe, so you could telephone the doctor's receptionist. Otherwise it may be simpler to go to a family planning clinic if your family doctor will not fit a diaphragm.

Clinics have the advantage that they carry out most diaphragm fittings and, as a result, are usually good at teaching how to insert the diaphragm, as well as experienced in judging sizes. They will also usually have stocks of the various sizes and of the spermicides. Many of the staff working in a clinic are women and if you would like to see a woman doctor you can ensure you do when making an appointment.

Whether you choose your family doctor or a clinic, the diaphragm and stocks of spermicide are free on prescription on the National Health Service.

Caps

This section should be read with the section on diaphragms. Because diaphragms are by far the more popular alternative, most of the information has been concentrated into that section, but much of it also applies to caps. Here we shall be concentrating on the differences.

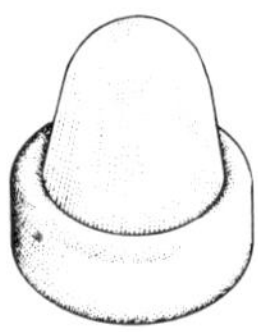

Cervical caps

Cervical caps are made of rubber. They are shaped roughly like a thimble and fit snugly over the cervix. Although in theory they fit more tightly than a diaphragm and so should be able to prevent sperm entering the cervical canal, it is usual to use them, too, with a spermicide. There are no formal statistics on their reliability on their own, but when used with a spermicide they are roughly as reliable as the diaphragm. The vimule and vault caps, described below, are basically variations on the plain cervical cap.

In Britain cervical caps have generally been used by women who have difficulty retaining a diaphragm, though Marie Stopes much preferred them and used them in her clinic. On the Continent, on the other hand, they were far more popular than diaphragms and very widely used until the advent of the Pill and the IUD.

They tend to be suitable only for some women. If the cervix is of the wrong shape or at the wrong angle, they will not fit properly or may be pushed off during intercourse.

The FPA-approved list gives only one cervical cap: the Prentif Cavity Ring, made by Lamberts (Dalston) Limited.

Sizes are measured by the internal diameter of the rim and range from 22 to 31 mm; the size chosen should match that of the base of the vaginal part of the cervix.

Before the cap is put on, a 5 cm strip of spermicide from the tube should be applied to each side of it and smeared over the surface. Alternatively, the bowl of the cap can be partially filled with 5 cm of spermicide cream or gel from a tube, the cap inserted and then a vaginal spermicide used.

A cervical cap is put in rim upwards and compressed between thumb and first finger. It is guided along the vagina until its back rim is just behind the cervix. Then it is pushed upwards on to the cervix where, if it is properly positioned, the cervix can be felt through it.

It has often been claimed that an advantage of the cervical cap is that it can be left in place throughout the month and only removed for menstruation. Indeed, a new cervical cap has been developed which can be left in place during menstruation because it has a small one-way flap which allows bleeding to pass. However, many experts are unhappy at the thought of blocking the uterine and vaginal secretions for long periods and until more research has been done it is recommended that the cervical cap be removed, like the diaphragm, about six hours after the last act of sex.

To remove the cap a finger is inserted under the rim and the cap is eased off. The Prentif has a hole in the rim for a thread to be attached, to make removal easier.

Cervical caps can be obtained free on prescription under the National Health Service along with their spermicides. They are neither made nor available in the United States, except in clinical trial centres approved by the Food and Drug Administration.

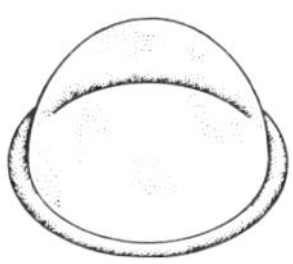

Vault cap

The vault cap is a dome made of rubber or plastic, and fits across the top end of the vagina, covering the cervix. It is held in place by suction (it has no metal rim). The air is expelled when it is pushed into place.

The FPA-approved list gives only one vault cap, the Dumas, made by Lamberts (Dalston) Limited. It ranges in size (measured by the outside diameter of the rim) from 50 to 75 mm, and the correct size is the smallest one which will fit evenly. It has roughly the same reliability as the diaphragm, if properly used.

Although it is not as easy to use as a diaphragm, it may be useful for women whose vaginal muscles are weak or whose cervix is split, torn or very short.

Before it is put in, a 5 cm strip of spermicide from the tube should be put on each side of the vault cap and smeared over the surfaces. It should not be smeared on the rim as suction would be reduced. Alternatively, the bowl of the cap can be partially filled with 5 cm of tubed spermicide, the cap inserted, and a vaginal spermicide used as well.

It is inserted in the same way as the cervical cap. It should be left in place for at least six hours after the last act of intercourse. While it is in place, straining downwards (for example, with a bowel movement) may dislodge it, so it is important to check that it has been pushed back into place.

To remove a vault cap, a finger is inserted under the rim to break the suction; the cap can then be withdrawn.

The vault cap has the same general advantages and disadvantages as the diaphragm.

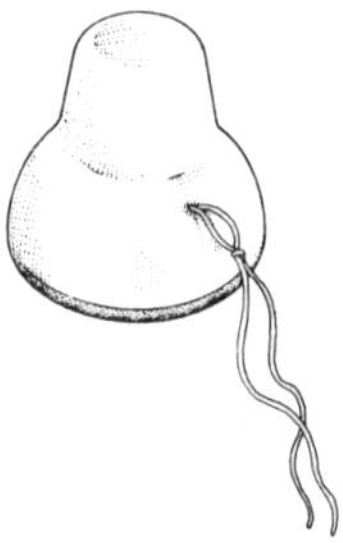

Vimule cap

The vimule cap is made of rubber and looks like a kind of hat with a deep brim. It fits over the cervix and the rim clings by suction to the vagina.

The FPA-approved list gives only one vimule cap, made by Lamberts (Dalston) Limited. It ranges in size (measured by the outside diameter of the rim) from 45 to 51 mm, and the correct size is the smallest one which will fit comfortably over the cervix and fit evenly into the vagina.

It may be useful for women who cannot hold other types of cap or diaphragm in place, especially those with a prolapse or cystocele (a hernia of the bladder projecting into the vagina).

The instructions for applying spermicide to the vimule cap, inserting it and removing it are the same for the other caps. Like the cervical cap, removal may be easier if a thread is attached to the rim: there is a hole there for the purpose.

Spermicides

The term 'spermicide' covers a range of products with several different ingredients. All of them are designed to be put into the vagina, as near the cervix as possible, and they act by killing or immobilising the sperm so that they cannot reach an egg. Some of them also form a kind of barrier over the cervix.

They may be supplied as aerosol foams, creams or jellies, or pessaries. Some pessaries should not be used with a diaphragm or cap because they may damage the rubber over time. Spermicides may also come in the form of foaming tablets or as a water-soluble plastic film.

Background

Although people have used all sorts of substances over the years to try to stop the sperm fertilising an egg – see 'Traditional Methods' – it was only in the 1930s that an attempt was made to standardise testing for spermicidal products and to get some idea of their real efficiency. Spermicides then became very popular, with a huge variety of brands and types being marketed, but interest in them fell rapidly with the development of the Pill and the IUD, and the number of products available today is comparatively small. Because most family planning programmes recommend that you use a spermicide in addition to barrier methods, it is likely that as the interest in diaphragms and condoms grows, interest in spermicides will revive too.

Safety

Modern spermicides are extremely safe to use, and their effects are largely local.

A few women – and sometimes their partners – used to find that some of the products caused irritation or slight soreness. This is less likely to happen with the spermicides available now, but if it does happen to you, try one with a different chemical base.

One excellent side effect of spermicides is that they reduce your chances of catching some sexually transmitted diseases or other vaginal infections. There is quite a lot of evidence that spermicides inhibit the growth, and the survival, of the bacterium which produces gonorrhoea. The evidence for spermicides having the same effect on trichomoniasis and candidiasis (thrush) is less good, but there is some, as there is also for spermicides having a protective effect against genital herpes.

Like condoms, diaphragms and caps, spermicides have not been studied with a fraction of the attention which the Pill and the IUD have had, so it is less easy to be certain that they have no other effects, though here again, given their popularity, any serious effect would probably have been noticed if there were one.

One area which does cause some concern is the possible effect of having used a spermicide if you do become pregnant. In theory, at least, it is possible that a sperm which got through and fertilised the egg could have been damaged by the spermicide on the way and if so the altered chromosomes might result in an abnormal embryo. Animal tests have not shown an increase in stillborn or deformed offspring, but one study of humans did suggest an increase in some particular types of congenital birth defect among the babies of spermicide-users. Unfortunately it was a study which raised more questions than it answered.

If you are using spermicides together with a condom or diaphragm the pregnancy rates are in any case very low.

Effectiveness

Used by themselves, spermicides have a quite high failure rate, or something under ten pregnancies for every hundred user-years. Used together with a diaphragm, cap or condom they are a very effective method. Caps and diaphragms in any case must be used with a spermicide, because part of the way they work is by holding the spermicide in place. They do need to be used according to the manufacturer's instructions though, which will be specific on points such as how long before intercourse you should insert them.

Spermicides deteriorate over time, or if their airtight containers are damaged so that they get damp or too hot. They should be stored in a cool place and preferably not kept for too long. In Britain, unless the spermicide packaging is damaged, with sensible storage you should be able to keep them for up to a year or so.

Acceptability

Because they are easy to buy and simple to use, spermicides have remained quite popular. With the exception of the aerosol foams, which are slightly more bulky, most of them are easy to carry around, and discreet. The soluble plastic film ones, which look like a sheet of gelatine, can be put over the penis or inserted straight into the vagina, which means they can be used by either a man or woman.

Some people find it inhibiting to have to break off love-making in order to put the spermicide in the vagina the right number of minutes before sexual intercourse. Others may find it difficult to get the timing right! (This can be especially difficult if you have sex more than once in quick succession.)

For some women – and some men – the greasiness or slipperiness which spermicides cause in the vagina reduces sensation, or is unaesthetic. For others, especially if the woman tends to vaginal dryness, spermicides can be quite helpful. The messiness of most spermicides is more noticeable in certain sexual positions, for example if the woman is on top.

Although their failure rate when used alone is not as low as that of many other contraceptives, spermicides make a good emergency measure, even on their own. With a condom, they are an easy contraceptive method for short-term use, for instance if you need extra temporary cover when starting the Pill, or because you have missed some Pills, or after you have come off the Pill before your periods are back to normal. Couples waiting after vasectomy for a final negative sperm count may also find them useful.

For casual sex, they have the advantage of limiting your chances of some sexually transmitted diseases – especially when used with a condom. But those who tend to be initially shy with a new partner may find that, like the condom, using a spermicide is difficult to do with nonchalance.

Availability

You can buy spermicides from any chemist. Though some people do not find it easy to ask for any contraceptive from a chemist, spermicides are now usually prominently displayed on a counter. You can also get your spermicides free on prescription if you are using a diaphragm or cap, and can pick them up from a family planning clinic.

You can also buy the spermicides for a cap by mail order, and Family Planning Sales Limited (whose profits go to the FPA) offer a twin pack (Two's Company) of condoms and spermicides for about £2 for ten of each, as well as a range of spermicides. Their own brand pessary – Double Check – costs under £1 for ten. There are reductions on larger orders.

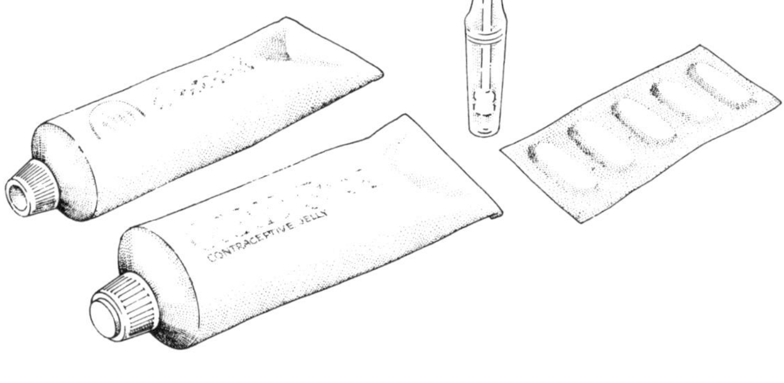

Different types of spermicides

Creams and jellies These are essential if you use a cap. The FPA-Approved List gives three brands of spermicidal jelly – Duragel made by LRC, Ortho-gynol Gel made by Ortho, and Staycept Jelly made by Syntex. Applicators for both the foams and the jellies are marketed by Ortho and by LRC.

Creams come in metal tubes, like the jellies, and the FPA-Approved List gives two – Duracreme from LRC and Orthocreme from Ortho. The approximate cost of a tube is just under £3.

Foams These come in aerosol containers. The FPA-Approved list gives Delfen, made by Ortho, and Emko Foam which is marketed by Syntex. Both have applicators, and cost a little under £5 (refills are about £4).

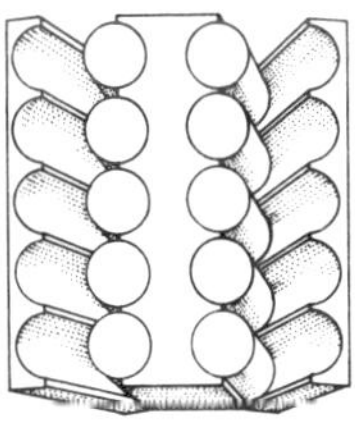

Pessaries These are small, bullet-shaped and slightly waxy; they come in individually sealed packs, or in plastic containers. The FPA-Approved List has three brands which can be used with diaphragms, caps and condoms: Orthoforms from Ortho; Staycept from Syntex; and Double Check from FPS. These cost up to about £2 for a dozen. Two more brands, Genexol and Rendells, both made by W. J. Rendell, should not be used with diaphragms or caps because over time they will cause the rubber to deteriorate. This should not affect their use with condoms, which are used only once.

Film This looks like a square of gelatine; one piece is either inserted into the vagina up to the cervix, or draped over the end of the penis. The only brand is called C-Film: it costs about £1 for ten squares.

The Pill

The Combined Pill

The combined oral contraceptive, intended to inhibit ovulation, is what most people mean when they talk about 'The Pill'. It is made up of two hormones, an oestrogen and a progestagen. Progestagens are chemical cousins of progesterone, which occurs naturally in the body, as do oestrogens. The Pill comes in the form of small tablets, usually in bubble packs with the days of the week printed against each tablet to make it easier to remember to take one. The pack may contain 21, 22 or 28 pills, depending on which type you use, and you take them for as many days of your monthly cycle as the pack provides for.

In order to understand how the Pill works, it helps if you first think about the female reproductive cycle as it is without hormonal contraception. If you are not on the Pill, in the first half of the monthly cycle before the egg is released from the ovary, the ovary itself produces only the hormone oestrogen, which is made within the follicles (clusters of cells). These have been activated by the follicle-stimulating hormone (FSH), which is produced by the pituitary at the base of the brain.

At mid-cycle, the luteinising hormone (LH) is released from the pituitary and causes the follicle to burst and release the egg. Once the follicle is empty, it begins to produce progesterone as well as oestrogen, and both hormones travel to the womb to thicken its lining so that it is prepared to receive a fertilised egg. After two weeks, if an egg has not been embedded in the lining of the womb, the ovaries stop producing oestrogen and progesterone, and the lining of the womb breaks down to be shed as menstrual blood.

If a fertilised egg has been embedded in the lining of the womb, another hormone is produced (by the embryo itself) which works on the follicles to ensure that they keep producing the oestrogen and progesterone needed for the lining of the womb to remain and provide nourishment for the foetus. Because the levels of oestrogen and progesterone remain high, the pituitary gets the message that there is no need to stimulate the ovaries again into producing more eggs. So the whole cycle goes into a stable state, with the pituitary producing much less FSH and LH and the follicles in the ovaries producing a steady trickle of oestrogen and progesterone instead of the surges around the different points of the cycle.

If, therefore, you take the Pill with doses of oestrogen and progestagen, so that there is a constant level of them in the system, the pituitary gets the same message that it would if you were pregnant. It stops triggering off the ovaries and the eggs are simply not released each month, so there is no menstrual cycle as such. However, because the effects of the hormones on the womb have been to build up the lining a little, if you stop taking the Pill for one week in each month this lining still comes away and there is some bleeding – called 'withdrawal bleeding'.

There is nothing particularly unusual about this: the Pill is producing the same results that your own hormones would be doing during the second half of the menstrual cycle, and throughout any pregnancy.

The only major difference is that the hormones are synthetic. Natural progesterone cannot be used because your digestive system will destroy it if you swallow it. The two synthetic oestrogens which are used in the Pill also work better than natural ones when taken by mouth.

Because the whole cycle is complicated, and the hormones involved affect the whole system, they work together as a contraceptive in more than one way. By inhibiting the pituitary from producing so much FSH, they stop the follicle from ripening and the egg from maturing. Because there is no surge of LH, no egg is released. The changes in the lining of the womb make it less suitable for the implantation of a fertilised egg, assuming that any egg could ever survive the previous two hurdles. The cervical mucus thickens slightly, which may prevent sperm getting through to an egg. It is also possible that the Fallopian tubes are affected so that any egg produced would find it more difficult to travel down towards the womb.

Background

There are around two and a half million women in Britain on the Pill, and about 65 million women round the world. It was invented in the 1950s, but only became generally available in Britain in 1961. Since then it must have become the most extensively investigated drug ever. This is partly because of the researchers' interest in the effects of a drug which acts throughout the whole body and which is taken by healthy women over a long period of time. Another likely reason for the research is many people's instinctive unease about its social effects: the Pill was the first 'modern' method – easy to use, discreet, reliable. It also distanced contraception from the act of sex. One way and another, it was seen as producing a social revolution – and it did.

Because of this, the findings of all the various studies have had a great deal more publicity than most medical research. In the Appendices we outline the different types of medical study which exist on contraception, and the kinds of questions you may want to ask in deciding on their value or importance.

There have been two particularly important British research projects on the Pill. One began in 1968 and is still being carried out by the Royal College of General Practitioners. It collected 23,600 women who used the Pill and 22,700 who did not, and set out to record and analyse all the medical conditions diagnosed for each woman by her family practitioner. The health of these women is still being followed.

The other study was carried out by the Family Planning Association and Oxford University. It included some 17,000 married women aged between 25 and 39 who used FPA clinics, and followed them during 1968–1975. Unlike the RCGP study, it did not have a control group of non-users whose family planning practice was not known. Instead, it compared Pill-users with users of two other contraceptive methods (diaphragm and IUD). Much of the information in this chapter is based on these two studies, which have been given world-wide recognition.

Early forms of the Pill had very much higher hormone levels than today's Pill. This resulted in more – and more serious – ill-effects being suffered by some women than seems to be the case with the 'second generation' Pills around now. Getting the dose right depends a bit on what you want from your contraceptive – where you put the dividing line between reliability and safety. In countries with automatic access to very early abortion, like China, women may be prepared to accept a slightly higher risk of contraceptive failure in return for reduced risk of ill-effects than they are when back-up abortion is more difficult. And the same woman, at different times in her life, may look at that equation quite differently. It is probably unlikely that the low-dose combined Pill could contain much lower hormone levels than it now does and still have its very high reliability. However, there are some alternatives to the traditional combined Pill – the triphasic Pill and the progestagen-only Pill – which some women may prefer (see later on in the section).

Safety

There are an enormous number of conditions, both good and bad, which have been associated with Pill use. We are concentrating on the most important ones and the ones which might affect quite a number of women. Obviously, if you suffer from any permanent illness or disability, both you and your doctor are going to know about it and think twice before deciding on any additional drug. Some women's medical history probably means they should not take the Pill at all – the conditions involved are listed under 'Reasons for not taking the Combined Pill'.

Most of the body changes or conditions which take place when you are on the Pill are the same ones that take place in pregnancy. If you have already had a baby, you may have some indication of whether or not any of the changes or conditions are likely to apply to you.

Possible good effects of Combined Pill use:

Menstrual cycle The Pill has a number of effects on the menstrual cycle and one of the most widely felt benefits for many women is a reduction of symptoms associated with their monthly cycle.

For a start, the Pill tends to regularise the cycle. You may find that even if your periods previously fluctuated wildly in timing, the Pill cycle of three weeks on and one week off leads to your withdrawal bleeding starting with clockwork regularity.

This evening-out of the hormonal pattern also tends to reduce some of the more tedious effects of irregular menstruation – increased body fluid, pre-menstrual tension, period pains and so on. There is usually less blood loss as well because it is not 'proper' menstrual bleeding. Besides being convenient, this also helps to decrease the possibility, or the severity, of anaemia – though this is less of a gain in Britain than in the Third World where a very high proportion of women are anaemic. The evening-out of the hormonal fluctuations in the body often seems to improve the skin, too, especially if you suffer from the kind of acne which is always worse before a period. (But only certain Pill combinations will help with this.)

Growths Use of the Pill also seems to reduce your chances of developing benign breast tumours and benign ovarian cysts. (Benign means that these growths are not cancers, but they can cause worry and problems even so, and often have to be operated on before you can be sure they are not serious.) There is some evidence which suggests that you are less likely to develop cancer of the ovaries or of the lining of the womb if you take the Pill – this may be the result of suppressed ovulation.

Some people argue, incidentally, that this suppression of ovulation is more 'natural' in a way than actually going through a monthly reproductive cycle. This is because in their pre-contraception state, most women in the past would have had comparatively few monthly cycles ending in menstruation: for most of their fertile years they would have been either pregnant or breastfeeding. If this was so, the argument goes, perhaps some more recent gynaecological conditions stem from modern women having too many monthly cycles. It is a theory which would be difficult to prove, and it has generally been greeted with some scepticism, although research is being carried out.

Pelvic inflammatory disease Pelvic infections are less common in Pill-users than in women using other contraceptive methods, or no method. The symptoms are primarily pelvic pain and tenderness, often with vaginal discharge, chills or fever. Although these infections are generally quite easily treated with antibiotics, women may fail to notice that they have one, or take any action about it even if they do. If untreated, pelvic infections can be a serious problem to women who have not yet had their families, as they can affect the Fallopian tubes and lead to sterility. It is not quite clear why Pill-users are less at risk but it seems that some of the changes in the body which the Pill causes have a protective effect.

Rheumatoid arthritis Fewer women who have used the Pill seem to suffer from rheumatoid arthritis, though again there does not seem to be much evidence about why they so not; in any case the protective effect seems fairly small.

Protection against pregnancy Above all, the most obvious benefit of the Pill is that it works. It is the most reliable method of preventing pregnancy, thus avoiding the choice between continuing a pregnancy, or asking for an abortion – which is itself not without risks, and which in any case is not a procedure anybody particularly wants to go through. Pregnancy carries its own risks, of course.

Ill-effects of Combined Pill use

The most important ill-effects of Pill use are those affecting the circulatory system. Thrombosis – the formation of a blood clot in veins or arteries – is more likely in Pill-users, just as it is in pregnancy. It is rare, and your chances of getting it if you are on the Pill are very small, but if you did develop a thrombosis it could be serious or even fatal (in the 35–39 age group there are four Pill-associated deaths per 100,000 women per year; the rate is very much lower for younger women).

Thrombosis in the veins Clotting in the deep veins of the legs was one of the first serious conditions to be linked with the Pill. Although it can happen to anybody, it is about four times more likely to happen to you if you take the Pill. It is occasionally fatal, but usually can be treated in hospital with drugs designed to thin the blood. Symptoms may include a painful and/or swollen leg and, if part of the clot breaks off and moves along the veins to the chest, a sharp – generally one-sided – pain in the chest, and perhaps some blood coughed up. When you stop taking the Pill, the extra risk drops to normal within two months.

Deep-vein thrombosis is also more common among people who are overweight, and those who have had recent operations and are confined to bed for a time. So if you are on the Pill and scheduled for an operation, or will have to spend a long time in bed, you should stop taking the Pill four to six weeks beforehand where possible. If you have acute appendicitis or have an accident, nobody is going to wait for a Pill-free month before treating you. But it is sensible to reduce the extra risk for planned surgery where you can.

Varicose veins are not the deep veins which tend to develop thrombosis and, unless you have had signs of a past thrombosis, or unless you are overweight, there is no reason why you should not choose the Pill as a contraceptive even if you have varicose veins. But if you developed any clotting, or phlebitis, you would have to change to another method in case a subsequent clot should be more serious.

Arterial thrombosis As you get older the walls of the arteries tend to roughen and slight clotting of the blood may occur on those roughened surfaces, blocking up the artery. This can result in a coronary thrombosis (heart attack) or a cerebral thrombosis (a kind of stroke). Strokes due to bleeding are also (rarely) associated with Pill use. These are things which can happen to anybody, and which have a number of contributory causes, including high blood cholesterol, and an increase in age, weight, high blood pressure and cigarette smoking. If you are over 35, and one or more of these factors applies to you, your chances of an arterial thrombosis are increased. If in addition you take the Pill, your risk rises again. The Pill has not been proved to increase the risk for women under 35, or for those women who do not have some of the other predisposing factors. Some of the factors themselves increase the risk more than taking the Pill does – for example, heavy cigarette-smoking.

High blood pressure Your blood pressure may rise slightly if you take the Pill. Some people, however, get a marked increase in blood pressure. While hypertension gives no symptoms and is seldom a serious problem on its own, it does seem to contribute to most of the diseases of the circulation, so needs to be watched. If there are any additional 'risk factors' – for example, if you are overweight or smoke – or if the blood pressure level rises considerably, it might be necessary to stop taking the Pill, or to change to a progestagen-only Pill (see later on in the section). Once you stop taking the Pill, your blood pressure normally returns to its usual level.

Less serious ill-effects

A number of other ill-effects have been attributed to the Pill although on some of them the actual evidence is poor.

Depression Depression is the commonest reason for giving up the Pill, although it is far from clear whether the Pill really causes it or whether there is simply a lot of depression around and people like to be able to tie it to something. (Remember what was said earlier about the Pill causing a social revolution? Not everybody finds that easy to take in their stride.) Some women find that taking extra Vitamin B_6 helps – its levels are lowered in the blood of some Pill-users – while others benefit from switching over to a Pill with a different hormone combination or a lower dose. If your doctor offers to treat your depression with anti-depressants or tranquillisers, though, it may be worth changing your method of contraception – at least for a three-month trial – instead of taking one drug to cancel the effects of another one. If you decide to continue the Pill *and* take anti-depressants or tranquillisers, check that the one you are given can be used together with your Pill (see the section on The Pill and other drugs).

Early symptoms Some women find, particularly in the first few months of Pill use, that they may get symptoms rather like those that many women experience in early pregnancy. These include nausea, dizziness, breast tenderness, fluid retention and/or slight weight gain, and breakthrough bleeding. Nausea and dizziness may be lessened if you take your Pill before going to sleep rather than in the morning. All of these minor but irritating symptoms should disappear if you carry on with the Pill: they tend to be most apparent in the first couple of months. If they do not, changing to a different hormone combination or a different dose will probably get rid of them. (Changing your dose does not, here, mean necessarily changing to a lower one – each woman's own hormone balance is slightly different, and it may be that you are getting too little oestrogen or progestagen to suit you.)

Effects of the Pill which may be good or bad

Some of the effects attributed to the Pill may be classed as a benefit or a drawback, depending on your own attitudes.

Menstrual cycle Because there is no real menstruation, the monthly bleeding – the shedding of the lining of the womb – is lessened. In some women, withdrawal bleeding stops altogether. This does not mean that you have become permanently infertile. Six months after stopping oral contraceptives, less than one per cent of those women who did not bleed regularly have not yet achieved regular periods. (There is a simple treatment to restore the cycle to that tiny percentage – i.e. changing Pill brands, especially to a phased oral contraceptive.)

For some women, monthly bleeding is important. They find it reassuring to know that they are not pregnant, and that their cycle is still continuing to function, or they just feel that such a monthly occurrence is 'normal'. Others – particularly if they have had a history of painful periods – may be glad to avoid them altogether, as may women athletes, or women whose religious beliefs place many taboos on their activities during a menstrual period. So whether you would be concerned if you found that on the Pill you had ceased to bleed depends very much on you.

Breast size Another possible effect of the Pill is to enlarge the breasts slightly. From the letters that go to the advice columnists in newspapers and magazines, it seems that few women are happy about their breasts, which they see as either too large or too small. If you think yours are too large, any further swelling (however tiny) might concern you. On the other hand, if you wish yours were larger, the Pill may help a little – but not much.

Libido (sex drive) Whether or not the Pill affects your sex drive seems to depend more on you than on the Pill itself. Some women – especially if they have tried another method of contraception which they have not liked very much – are so pleased with the spontaneity of love-making which the Pill offers, and with the relaxation from worry about a possible pregnancy, that their sex drive actually increases. Others may find that precisely because it is so reliable, they lose interest in sex because there is hardly a possibility that it will result in a pregnancy. A few women may find that there is a slight lessening of vaginal lubrication on the Pill: this can be helped by the use of a lubricant jelly.

Return of fertility Although the Pill is unlikely to make you infertile, it may delay slightly the time taken to get pregnant when you come off it. In any group of women who are not using the Pill, it will normally take from six months to a year for 80-90 per cent of them to become pregnant.

With Pill-users, the timespan may be a little longer, but by the end of about two years they are as likely to be pregnant as any other woman. Again, whether that matters to you will depend on your plans and how urgently you want a baby after stopping the Pill. On balance, it may be a benefit that there could be this delay. Many doctors now recommend that you don't try to get pregnant immediately you come off the Pill, but use another method for three months to make sure that your own hormonal mechanisms are working normally.

Reasons for not taking the Combined Pill

Having said all this, there are a few conditions which you might have or have had which mean that you should not use the Pill. These include breast or vaginal tract cancer; deep-vein thrombosis; heart attack or angina; any sort of stroke; abnormal vaginal bleeding (if the cause is undiagnosed); and focal migraine. Focal migraine is a very unusual and specific type: check with your doctor if you are not sure which sort of migraine you have. There is no reason why most migraine sufferers should not use the Pill – some people find the Pill makes the migraines worse, others that it improves them.

Other conditions which make it unlikely that the Pill would be a good choice for you are a high blood cholesterol level; severe diabetes; high blood pressure; overweight (if you are more than 50 per cent above what is right for your height); age (if you are over 35); and the habit of heavy smoking (say, 15 or more cigarettes a day). But remember, the biggest single risk to your health from those four factors is the one from smoking.

Effectiveness of the Combined Pill

Taken every day according to instructions, the Pill is the most reliable method of contraception, with a failure rate as low as 0.1 per cent. In practice, as is true for all methods, the failure rate is a little higher. There are several things which may interfere with its efficiency.

Starting the Pill You should not assume that you are covered against risk as soon as you begin your first pack of Pills. This is only true in certain circumstances.

The standard instruction when you begin taking the Pill is to wait until your period starts (day 1 of your cycle), and take the first Pill on the fifth day and one a day thereafter. However, if, during that particular month, you have a very short cycle, the follicle may already have begun to ripen. So much oestrogen may have been produced that it would be too late for the Pill to damp down the LH that this triggers and stop the release of an egg. If you do begin taking the Pill on this schedule, you must use another method as well for at least the first 14 days after you begin the Pill.

A more recently developed technique is to take your first Pill on the first day of your period, and one a day thereafter. You will have a short cycle in the first month, of course, but after that it should settle down to a normal 28 days. With this method you will tend to have more breakthrough bleeding in the first month, but as far as is known this technique is reliable – in other words you will not have to depend on an additional method at first.

Missing a Pill However methodical you are, sooner or later you may forget to take a Pill at the right time or on the right day. Obviously it makes more sense to take a Pill approximately 24 hours after the last one – for example, just before going to bed each night – but, if you miss one and remember within the next 12 hours, take the missed one immediately and the next one at its normal time. If you have forgotten for more than 12 hours, take the missed Pill immediately and the next one at its normal time, but use an additional method of contraception for the next 14 days – regardless of when during the month the Pill was missed, and regardless of whether you get either breakthrough bleeding or your normal withdrawal bleeding. In short, if you have missed a Pill for more than 12 hours, use an additional method for two full weeks.

If you have missed more than one Pill, take two Pills at

once and then the one for that day at its usual time, and finish the pack normally. But for the next two weeks, consider yourself unprotected and use an additional method of contraception. If you had intercourse during that time when you had forgotten the Pills, you may wish to consider postcoital contraception (see the section on this.) At the end of the month, if there is no withdrawal bleeding, you should go and see a doctor – but continue your Pill routine along with an additional method because (as we have already explained) not everybody gets withdrawal bleeding each month. It does not necessarily mean that you are pregnant.

Stomach upsets or vomiting Diarrhoea and vomiting can both result in the Pill being flushed out of the body instead of absorbed into the system. They probably account for most of the accidental pregnancies while on the Pill.

If you vomit within four hours of taking a Pill, take another as soon as you think you can keep it down. If it is taken within 12 hours, and stays down, you will probably be protected. So that you do not get muddled over the days, or end up one Pill short, it makes sense to take the extra one from a different pack – and to keep the rest of that pack for future emergencies. (If you take biphasic or triphasic Pills, remember to take the spare Pill from the right group.) If you are already on your last pack and cannot do this, remember to go and get another prescription before the end of the month so that you do not have a short month.

Should the second – replacement – Pill you take also be vomited, go back to the rest of the month's Pills only when your stomach has settled, but use an additional method for the next 14 days, and regardless of the time of the month when you missed some, and regardless of whether you bleed or not. A Pill which was taken more than four hours before you vomited should have been absorbed.

While you have an attack of diarrhoea, you should assume that the Pills have not been absorbed. Go on taking them according to the usual routine, but use an additional method of contraception until 14 days after the attack, again regardless of the time of the month when the diarrhoea happened or of any bleeding.

In view of how easy it is to lose a Pill, and taking into account the occasions when you vomit or have a stomach upset, it seems a pity that Pill manufacturers do not provide spares. An extra Pill with each pack – in a separate bubble clearly marked 'Spare' or 'Duplicate', provided in the same way that many firms provide an extra button for clothes – would be a useful innovation.

The Pill and other drugs Many drugs tend to interact with each other as well as on the body. Some drugs can interfere with the effects of the Pill and may minimise its contraceptive value. Perhaps the most common group is antibiotics. Exactly how big a risk they are for most Pill-users is not altogether clear because if you are ill enough to be needing antibiotics your sexual activity is likely to be reduced too – but women who are taking the Pill because of its high reliability would probably rather be safe than sorry. In which case, if you are given a course of ampicillin (e.g. Penbritin), amoxycillin (Amoxil), or tetracyclines, you should use an additional method during the course and for 14 days afterwards.

Some drugs used to treat arthritis – phenylbutazone (Butazolidin) and oxyphenbutazone (Tanderil; Tandacote) – may also lessen the effect of the Pill. So too may barbiturates, sedatives and tranquillisers such as chlorpromazine (Largactil) and memprobamate (Equanil; Milonorm). Drugs used in the treatment of epilepsy are particularly thought to interfere with the Pill's effect. If you are put on a course of any of these you should use an additional method while on that course and for 14 days afterwards. If you are taking any of them long-term, you may have to discuss the use of an alternative contraceptive method, or perhaps of a stronger type of Pill.

This is not a complete list of drugs which may affect the efficiency of the Pill. More are being found gradually and it is possible that even drugs you can buy without a prescription from a chemist may influence the Pill. If you get breakthrough bleeding while taking any drug, consult your doctor or a family planning clinic.

Finally, changing from a higher to a lower dose may also affect the Pill's contraceptive value. Your body will no longer be getting the same level of hormonal messages so the pituitary might begin to trigger off the release of an egg. If you begin the new lower-dose pack, without waiting for withdrawal bleeding, there is no need for extra protection. You may have some breakthrough bleeding during the changeover month, especially in the first few days, but it can be ignored. At the end of the first 21 lower-dose Pills, you have your usual seven-day break and bleeding, and then carry on as usual.

Acceptability of the Combined Pill

The Pill is very easy to use: you simply swallow one a day for three weeks and have one week off before starting again. If you prefer to take something every day in a settled routine instead, you can opt for one of the brands which has a lactose supplement (see 'The 28-day Pill').

It is relatively discreet to use, and it should not be difficult to keep the fact that you are on the Pill to yourself, if you want to. It is also easy to carry around if you are going away for a few days, for example.

Pills don't deteriorate very easily, though they can if the pack gets damaged and damp gets in. But you should be able to keep up to a year's supply without any problems of damage.

They are also one of the safest drugs to have around the home. An overdose of the contraceptive Pill is one of the very few drugs which will do nobody any harm; if a small child swallows your whole pack he or she may be sick and, if the child is a girl, she may have a little bleeding from the vagina – but there will be no permanent harm.

When the Pill first became available, doctors used to suggest that women taking it should come off it every two years for a few months. This was logical at the time – after all, it was a new drug and nobody was sure about its long-term effects – but it was often annoying for the user, and it is now generally agreed that there is no advantage in coming off it unless you want a baby or unless there are medical reasons for stopping it altogether. Many older women, however, who have completed their families, are not very keen on continuing to take a drug for a long period of time.

For most women, the Pill is a safe and convenient method of contraception. But it, and its derivatives (injectables and implants), are the only contraceptive method which rely on hormones which affect your whole system, so many women have worries about it, even while they are using it. This can mean that they tend to link any health worries they have with the Pill. They may assume, for example, that an increased number of headaches must be caused by the Pill, without checking the other possible causes – their eyesight, or the lighting in the new office they are working in, or a personal unhappiness or tension.

For a minority of women who loathe taking any drug for any reason, and would rather suffer pain than take an aspirin, even, the Pill is probably not a sensible choice of contraceptive. They are unlikely ever to be at ease with it.

But a steady two and a half million women in Britain each year do take the Pill, and for them it is a question of putting the risks and the benefits into context. Every drug in the world has side effects; some of the ones you can buy over the counter, without prescription, are more likely to cause serious ill-effects and even death, than the Pill.

There are, of course, still unanswered questions about the Pill – for example, its effects on future generations and on very young users. These questions cannot, for obvious reasons, be answered for many years.

Young Pill-users Teenagers have been taking the Pill since the early 1960s, but should very young ones do so? There is no evidence that giving very young girls the Pill is harmful, but nevertheless there are doubts about interfering with the very complex hormonal system until it has had time to get properly established. So the Pill is probably not a particularly good method for a girl before her periods have become regular.

There is another area of doubt, too: breast cancer has been linked with some oestrogens. Breast cancer is the commonest cancer in women, and there have been a number of studies to see if the Pill could, because of its oestrogen content, affect a woman's chances of getting it. So far there is no clear evidence either that taking the Pill makes you more or less likely to get breast cancer (though, as we said – see 'possible good effects of Pill use' – you are less likely to get non-cancerous breast growths if you have used the Pill). Breast cancer tends to be most common in women after the 'change of life', so it will not really be until a large number of women have been studied over a very long time that we will know whether or not the Pill makes any difference. Again, girls starting the Pill when very young could be at greater risk.

On the other hand, an unwanted pregnancy in a very young girl is probably the biggest tragedy of all, and the risks of pregnancy itself to a girl under 16 are very much higher than those to an adult woman. If she is having sex and is unable or unwilling to use barrier methods each time, then the Pill might be her only option. (An IUD is unlikely to be suitable, because of the risk of pelvic inflammatory disease.) The situation for under-16s is complicated because of the legal position too: see the 'Availability' section.

The Pill and babies Another area of worry for many women is whether the Pill might harm the babies they have later. Over the last 20 years, a number of studies have found that ex-Pill-users do not have more spontaneous abortions (miscarriages) than women who have never used it, nor have they found more abnormalities in the babies born to previous Pill-users. But it makes sense to wait after coming off the Pill until you have had at least one proper menstrual bleeding before you try to get pregnant. This way you can be sure at least when the baby was conceived, and count the months of pregnancy properly. You would, of course, have to use an alternative contraceptive method between coming off the Pill and the first proper period. Some people recommend that you leave a rather longer gap between coming off the Pill and getting pregnant, and if you prefer to do this, you should use an alternative method for three months.

It can happen – though rarely – that you take the Pill by mistake once you are already pregnant. This is so rare that even the biggest studies of the Pill have not found many cases to go on, certainly not enough for anybody to say definitely whether there could be an effect on the foetus. So far there is no proof that it makes any difference to the outcome of pregnancy, either in terms of making you more likely to lose the baby, or of its being born with a defect.

The Pill and breastfeeding Once the baby is born, some doctors believe that you should not use a combined Pill until the baby is weaned. Using the Pill reduces the amount of breast-milk and the length of time that breast-milk goes on being produced. This is not true of the progestagen-only Pill (see overleaf) which does not seem to suppress the quantity of breast-milk or shorten the time it lasts. If you have found the Pill a useful and convenient method of contraception, and would prefer to continue to use it after having a baby, you should switch to a progestagen-only Pill (see below) while you are breastfeeding. Again, a number of studies have looked at the effects on the baby getting tiny amounts of synthetic hormones through the breast-milk, and no harmful effects have been found, though to be certain we would probably have to wait for a couple of generations.

The 28-day Pill

This is an ordinary combined oestrogen and progestagen Pill but it comes in a pack with seven extra pills of a different colour. For 21 days you take the combined Pill, followed by a lactose (a sugar) pill for the remaining seven days. It is designed to help those women who find it easier to remember a daily routine if it is not broken up every three weeks.

In some countries, especially in the Third World, the seven non-contraceptive tablets contain vitamins and/or iron as a supplement to the woman's diet. This is not so in Britain, where severe under-nourishment and vitamin deficiency or anaemia are less common.

The Progestagen-only Pill, or 'Mini-Pill'

The progestagen-only Pill contains a lower dose of progestagen than most combined Pills, and also, as its name suggests, no oestrogen. This small dose is probably not enough to stop the follicles ripening and the egg maturing, and it does not always stop the LH increasing enough to trigger off the release of an egg (in fact, it only stops about one in two eggs being released). However, it is sufficient to cause the mucus at the entrance to the cervix to become thicker and much more difficult for the sperm to penetrate, so during the months when an egg is released, it is much less likely for the sperm to get to it.

In about half of the cycles the LH does rise, and an egg is released, and then the rest of the cycle takes place as though you were not using a hormonal contraceptive, so many of the monthly bleedings will be normal periods and not withdrawal bleedings.

The progestagen-only Pill has fewer side-effects than the combined Pill, and it may therefore be a good alternative for women who find that even the lowest dose of oestrogen in the combined Pill upsets them, as well as for older women who want to avoid the risks of the combined Pill which increase with age. The progestagen-only Pill does not interfere with the amount of breast-milk you produce, or how long the breast-milk lasts, so it can be a suitable contraceptive if you are breastfeeding a baby.

Unfortunately, it also has a much higher failure rate than the combined Pill. The rate is between 0.5 and 4 per hundred woman-years. Quite a number of those failures result from people forgetting to take it each day, or not taking it at the same time of day. It must be taken every morning, without fail, and throughout your periods as well. It tends to produce quite a lot of irregular and break-through bleeding, which can be a nuisance to some women and a real drawback to women whose religion imposes taboos on their activities while bleeding.

The progestagen-only Pill is used by far fewer women than those who use the ordinary combined Pill, and it is also newer, so that less is known about its possible effects – although it is generally agreed that there are probably fewer ill-effects. However, one is that if you do get pregnant while on the progestagen-only Pill, the pregnancy is more likely to be ectopic. The same is true of the IUD. The probable reason, in both cases, is that because the lining of the womb is less receptive to an egg being implanted, a fertilised egg which gets to the womb may be rejected. But an egg which attaches itself to the Fallopian tube (and fertilised eggs do this from time to time) might survive. It is not clear whether the progestagen-only Pill actually makes it more likely that an egg will develop in the Fallopian tube, or whether the rate of tubal pregnancies is the same as in the rest of the population but that the counter-balancing ones which would otherwise occur in the womb are mostly prevented.

On the whole, the progestagen-only Pill is probably of most value to specific groups of women – the very young, those breastfeeding, women over 35, or those who for one or another reason should not use an ordinary combined Pill, but like oral contraception.

Triphasic and Biphasic Pills

These are a new version of combined oral contraceptives, in which the dosages of oestrogen and progestagen are varied during the month. In the triphasic Pill pack, there are three lots of Pills, each group coloured differently, and having a different combination of the two hormones. It is essential that the Pills are taken in the right order. Biphasic Pills – only available in Britain from 1982 – are packs containing two lots of pills. The first seven contain less progestagen than the remaining ones. Both types attempt to mimic more closely the hormone fluctuations in a normal cycle.

Triphasics are also new – they went on the British market during the second half of 1980 – and medical opinion at the moment is that if you are happy on an ordinary combined Pill, there is no advantage in changing to a triphasic, but that if you have some problems with the combined Pill, triphasics may help because they have a lower overall dose of progestagen than any of the others. For instance, the lower progestagen dose could help to limit the development of hypertension.

Tricyclic Pills

As we describe in the section 'Effects of the Pill which may be good or bad', some women want to avoid monthly periods altogether, and a few researchers argue that this may be 'natural'. So there are trials going on of ordinary combined Pills taken every day, with one seven-day bleeding period every third month. Given in this way, combined Pills have been nicknamed 'tricyclic'. We still do not have any real information about the benefits and risks of taking the Pill in that way (although, obviously, over three months you will be getting a third more of the oestrogen and progestagen than you would in the normal 21-day on, 7-day off, cycle). It is improbable that your doctor would agree to give you the extra Pills to do this except as part of a trial.

Sequential Pills

Sequential Pills are no longer available in Britain, or in many other countries. Sequential Pill packs consisted of oestrogen on its own for the first 14–16 days, followed by tablets containing both oestrogen and progestagen for the next 5–7 days,with seven Pill-free days before the next cycle. The dose of oestrogen used was very high and despite this there was a quite high failure rate.

Availability

There is a wide variety of Pills available in Britain. The FPA-Approved List gives eight low-oestrogen-dose brands and fourteen medium-oestrogen-dose ones, as well as three low-oestrogen and low-progestagen triphasic brands and six progestagen-only Pills. One of the low-oestrogen preparations, and two of the medium-oestrogen ones, as well as one of the triphasics, is a 28-day pack containing 21 Pills and seven lactose tablets or placebos.

Although the Pill is available free of charge on a National Health Service prescription, there is a considerable difference in price between brands of Pill, and your GP may be unwilling to prescribe, or your clinic stock, some brands unless there is a good medical reason. Most family practitioners will prescribe the Pill – in fact, most Pill-users get them from their doctors rather than a clinic. If yours will not, you can get a list from a post office or your local Family Practitioner Committee of other local practitioners who will see contraceptive clients not signed up with them.

Depending on your doctor's views and his knowledge of you, he may or may not give you a physical examination when you ask for the Pill, with further examinations at intervals while you are on it. Alternatively, a nurse attached to the practice may do so. If you go to a family planning clinic, you will be given a physical examination, including breast examination and a cervical smear, again by a doctor or nurse. Even if there is no examination you should insist on having your blood pressure taken.

Having a cervical smear from time to time (how often depends on your age and lifestyle, and should be discussed with a doctor) is good preventive medicine, and so too is a breast examination. It has, however, nothing to do with the Pill itself and if you do not want to link the two things, then there is no reason why you should. If you dislike having a full examination when you go for your prescription, you will probably find that your family practitioner makes less of a fuss over a routine visit.

On the other hand, if you have any problems or worries about the Pill, or develop any symptoms which you think may be linked to its use, you might prefer to go to a clinic where the staff specialise in contraception. It depends on your relationship with your doctor. You may also prefer to go to a clinic if you would rather see a woman doctor, because most family planning clinic doctors are women and you can certainly ask in advance for an appointment with a woman doctor there.

Convenience is another question: most people's doctors have a surgery closer to them than a family planning clinic, and their doctor may well be able to offer them an appointment more quickly, and at shorter notice, than many clinics can do.

Anonymity can be an advantage if you are single and want the Pill, and that is more likely if you go to a clinic than to your family doctor. A clinic doctor may also be less likely to moralise – though this is not necessarily true and there are plenty of sympathetic GPs around, especially among the younger ones.

If you are under 16 your partner will be breaking the law by having sex with you. But the law does not prevent a doctor from prescribing contraceptives for you if he or she feels that it is in your best interests not to get pregnant. Here you may find a clinic doctor more sympathetic than your own GP. But whichever one you go to will encourage you to tell your parents that are using contraception, and they may offer to help you do this. They should not tell your parents without your permission. If you do not want to tell your parents, the doctor may still decide to give you the Pill, but it may be with considerable reluctance.

Apart from personal preferences, there is no particular reason why either a clinic or a family practitioner is a 'better' place to go for the Pill. Unfortunately, very few of the potentially serious ill-effects of the Pill can be forecast accurately in advance. Wherever you go, you should insist on having your blood pressure taken regularly, because that will help in checking that you are not at risk over the circulatory dangers associated with the Pill. Wherever you go, if you are over 35, overweight and/or a smoker, you will probably be advised to use another method. Apart from these exceptions, however, if you are a healthy woman with no particular medical history, nobody can say in advance that you are not suited to Pill use.

So why see a doctor at all? In many countries the Pill is not a prescription drug, and non-medical people have been trained to ask basic questions to check the health of the woman and to take her blood pressure – and to refer her to a doctor if she has any problems. In Britain, efforts to make the Pill more easily available led to the setting up by the Department of Health and Social Security of a Joint Working Group to look at making the Pill more widely available. It reported in 1976 that the Pill should remain on prescription, but that for many women it did not need a doctor to prescribe it, or even a 'professional' person, just somebody with appropriate training.

It is true that in some family planning clinics nurses now dispense the Pill, but the idea behind widening distribution – that many consumers would prefer to get their contraceptives without going to a clinic or doctor – has been ignored. You still cannot go to your local chemist, say, or your social worker, and pick up the Pill. Arrangements have foundered

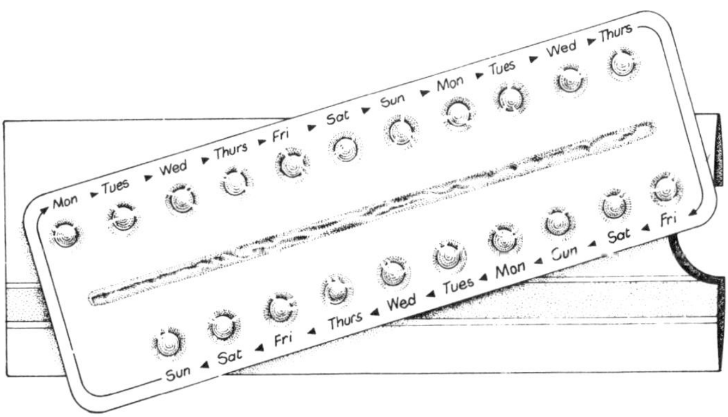

on politics (including the medico-legal aspects) – both between the various professional bodies concerned, and government reluctance to get involved – and on money. Meanwhile the choice for the individual consumer remains restricted when there is no good health reason for that restriction.

Conclusions

The Pill remains one of the easiest methods of contraception to use, as well as the most reliable. For most healthy women, it is also a generally safe method. It should be avoided if you have blood pressure problems, or if you are over 35 or overweight or smoke more than 15 cigarettes a day (though, if you like the Pill, it would make more sense to give up smoking!).

Apart from the sheath it is probably the best method for a young woman or one with various sexual partners. (A very young girl, though, should think carefully before going on the Pill.) It may be less suited to women who are older, have completed their families or who just don't like the idea of taking a drug. It is less easy to get hold of than the sheath – though no more difficult than the cap or IUD – and there are times, such as during and after an upset stomach, when an additional method will be needed as well. It will not affect your chances of having a baby, or the health of that baby, though it may slightly delay the time it takes you to get pregnant. The possible ill-effects cannot generally be foreseen for a particular woman, but in any case they are quite rare; the benefits, though less dramatic, tend to be more widespread.

Injectable contraceptives

There are various sorts of injectable contraceptives in use or under trial around the world, but the best-known one in Britain is a synthetic progestagen. This is injected into the arm or buttock, every two or three months, depending on which progestagen is used. The injectable contraceptive is not very different from the progestagen-only Pill, except that it is injected rather than swallowed and is absorbed over time, instead of daily.

In the first half of the monthly cycle, until the egg is released from the ovary, the ovary itself produces only the hormone oestrogen, which is made within the follicles. These have been stimulated into action by the follicle-stimulating hormone (FSH) produced by the pituitary at the base of the brain.

At mid-cycle, the luteinising hormone (LH) is released from the pituitary and triggers off the bursting of the follicle to release the egg. Once the follicle is empty, it begins to produce progesterone as well as oestrogen, and both hormones travel to the womb to thicken its lining so that it is prepared to receive a fertilised egg. After two weeks, if an egg has not been embedded in the lining of the womb, the ovaries stop producing oestrogen and progesterone and the lining of the womb breaks down and is shed in the form of menstrual blood.

If you take progestagen (a synthetic version of progesterone) throughout the month, you will obviously interfere with this cycle: because it is present at the beginning of the cycle, the pituitary fails to get the message that the previous cycle has been completed, so it is less likely to produce the usual amount of FSH. This, in turn, means that the follicle is less likely to ripen fully and an egg be released.

Mcanwhilc, thc progcstagcn has had somc of thc othcr effects which it would produce normally only in the second part of the cycle. In particular, it has caused the mucus at the entrance to the cervix to become much thicker, and more difficult for the sperm to penetrate, so that even if an egg is released it is much more difficult for the sperm to get at it.

Changes in the lining of the womb make it less well suited to the implantation of a fertilised egg. The Fallopian tubes may also be affected so that any egg produced would find it more difficult to travel towards the womb.

Background

The first injectable became available for contraception in the second half of the 1960s but they continue to be a controversial method for a number of reasons. Some of these are discussed later in the chapter. A further area of criticism is that injectables are 'dumped' in third world countries but banned in the West. A large number of Western countries do in fact use injectables, but the best-known and most widely used one – depot medroxyprogestarone acetate (DMPA, Depo-Provera, or Depo) – is not approved for use in the United States. At the moment, it is approved in Britain for short-term use only (for those women who have just had rubella vaccination against German measles and for couples where the man is waiting for clear sperm counts after a vasectomy) although the Committee on the Safety of Medicines recommended extending that approval. Also approved in Britain for short-term use is Noristerat made by Schering. Doctors have wide discretion in prescribing drugs, though, and may offer either in other circumstances.

The reasons for the ban in the United States are not altogether clear. The American Food and Drug Administration (FDA) works through advisory committees of specialists, which recommended that DMPA should be approved as a contraceptive. The FDA rejected their advice.

DMPA continues to be widely used in America as a treatment for cancer of the womb, and, as American doctors have a similar discretion in prescribing drugs as their British colleagues, some continue to give it as a contraceptive.

This particular injectable has been approved as a contraceptive both by the World Health Organisation and by the International Planned Parenthood Federation.

Safety

Of the two hormones in the combined Pill, it is the oestrogen which is responsible for most of the serious ill-effects, especially those on the circulatory system. Injectables, like the progestagen-only Pill, are designed to avoid those effects.

Irregular bleeding Much the most common ill-effect of injectables, like the progestagen-only Pill, is that they interfere with the normal bleeding pattern. Your cycle may be disrupted, and you may have break-through spotting or bleeding during the cycle. Some women find that their monthly bleeding is much heavier, but more of them tend to stop bleeding altogether. About a third of DMPA-users will cease to have any monthly bleeding by the end of a year. (Any bleeding is less likely to be true menstruation than in the case of the progestagen-only Pill. The dose of progestagen is higher in an injectable and it seems probable that a smaller proportion of the eggs ripen fully or are released into the womb.)

This irregular bleeding pattern, or the absence of bleeding, does not seem to affect your chances of having a baby later, although it may slightly delay the time you take to get pregnant. After 18 months, you are as likely to have conceived as if you are an ex-combined Pill user.

Some women find the absence of any bleeding a benefit, especially if menstruation limits their activities, or if they have previously suffered painful periods, or are likely to be anaemic. Others like to feel that their body is continuing to tick over normally, and to be able to check that they have not become pregnant.

Much more upsetting may be irregular bleeding and spotting. This can be a real drawback for women whose culture or religion limits their activities when they are bleeding, and it may increase anaemia (though this is less of a problem in Britain than in countries where many women are under-nourished and have frequent pregnancies). Most women find their menstrual cycles return to normal within six months of their last injection.

Weight gain You may gain some weight while using an injectable contraceptive. In most cases this should be no more than a few pounds: if there is a noticeable or rapid weight gain, you should check with your doctor.

Effects in pregnancy and on babies There is much less risk of becoming pregnant while using an injectable than there is with the progestagen-only Pill, both because the dose is somewhat higher and is therefore more likely to stop a ripe egg being released, and because many of the 'failures' of the progestagen-only Pill are the result of failure to take it on time.

To make sure that you are not already pregnant without knowing it when you begin to use an injectable, you will usually be asked to have your first injection during the first seven days of your cycle.

If you come off DMPA in order to have a baby you should wait until your periods are completely back to normal before trying to start one. So far there is no evidence that any residual progestagen left in the body when you stop taking the drug has any adverse effect on the baby's health, but – as with any drug – it makes good sense to be absolutely certain that it is out of your system before getting pregnant.

Like progestagen-only Pills, injectables do not affect the quantity of milk produced when breastfeeding, or the time that breastfeeding can last. There is no evidence so far that the small amounts of the hormone which are transferred to the baby in breast-milk have any ill-effects, though as we said about the Pill, it will take some generations before we can be absolutely certain of the long-term effects.

Breast tumours Breast tumours have been found in beagle dogs given very high doses of DMPA, but this is not very helpful as beagles produce the same results with all sorts of progestagens – including the natural progesterone – so scientists no longer place much reliance on tests using them. Studies in humans have not shown any increase in breast tumours or cancer among users of DMPA.

Cancer of the lining of the womb Again, scientists have

found a small number of cases of cancer of the lining of the womb among monkeys given huge doses of DMPA for a long period, but it is not clear what this means for humans. There have been no similar cases among the women who have used it, though research is still going on. DMPA is widely used as a drug to treat cancer of the womb, as well as for contraceptive purposes, but while it seems unlikely that it actually causes cancer of the lining of the womb, it may be that it does not always prevent it.

Reversibility The big difference between an injectable and most other forms of contraception is that you cannot stop it instantly. If you are one of the people who suffer unpleasant effects with an injectable, you are stuck with them for the next three months and perhaps rather longer, because the drug does not stop acting at the end of its three-month dose, but diminishes over the next few days. If you decide to use an injectable, you should be prepared to accept any possible effects for the period the drug will last.

Acceptability

Unless there is really strong medical evidence that you should avoid using a particular contraceptive method, the decision about which to use should always be yours alone. Doctors and others can advise on the different possibilities but it is you who must choose for yourself. Because an injectable is irreversible until the effect wears off, it is all the more important that you make the decision.

Doctors spend most of their time making judgements about which drugs to give a sick patient, and some of them are not so good at resigning that decision-making when it comes to a healthy woman's choice of contraceptive. However, if a doctor gives you the Pill when you are not convinced the Pill is for you, you can throw the pack away. Even if he inserts an IUD you don't want, for example after an abortion, you can go elsewhere and have it removed immediately. This is not the case with injectables.

There have been instances when women have been given

injectables without proper explanation and even without knowing what they were getting. This is bad medical practice and indefensible. It is not a sensible reason, though, to criticise the contraceptive itself, any more than it is a reason for distrusting the whole medical profession.

Injectables may be a good method of contraception if you want something with high reliability (they are second only to the Pill, with a failure rate of well below one per hundred woman-years) but are not prepared to accept, or are unable to tolerate, the oestrogen-related risks of the combined Pill. You may find a three-monthly injection less of a bind than the meticulous daily routine of the progestagen-only Pill. For some women, the high probability of ceasing to bleed while using an injectable is quite an advantage; others, who may get intermittent bleeding or spotting, may be less enthusiastic.

Using an injectable is absolutely discreet, and there is nothing you have to remember to carry about or do. It could be a good method if you are breastfeeding because it doesn't reduce breast-milk, or if you are over 35 or smoke or are overweight and don't want to continue on the Pill.

It could also be a good method if your sex life is rather erratic, because it gives constant protection without effort and without either the oestrogen-related Pill risks or the higher risk of pelvic inflammatory disease with an IUD.

By far its biggest drawback is the interference with your menstrual cycle, and the fact that whatever the side effects you must endure them for as long as the drug lasts.

Availability

As we have said, at the moment there are no injectables generally available in Britain. The Committee on the Safety of Medicines approved DMPA – trade name Depo-Provera (an Upjohn Pharmaceuticals product) – for wider use in early 1982 but the Health Minister overruled the Committee, so it remains available only for short-term use by women who have just had rubella vaccine against German measles, and for couples where the man has just had a vasectomy and is waiting for the tests to show he is no longer fertile. Individual doctors, including family practitioners, hospital doctors and some family planning clinic doctors, do offer DMPA among the methods they are willing to prescribe. In any case the injectable is only available on prescription, but is free under the NHS.

If you decide you would like to use DMPA, your choice of where to get it is currently pretty limited – it would be a question of finding somebody who was prepared to prescribe it, rather than choosing which provider to use. If you are lucky enough to have a choice, you will have to weigh the possibly greater expertise of a specialist clinic against the greater convenience of going to your local GP, because you will have to go every two or three months for the injection.

Once you have been seen by a doctor, there is no reason why the injections he prescribes cannot be dispensed by a nurse. In many countries injectables are given by people with very limited training, entirely satisfactorily. You may be given an internal examination and a cervical smear before being given an injectable, especially if you go to a clinic – there is no intrinsic reason why you should be, although it is good general preventive medicine. If you really dislike having these things done you can ask to skip them.

Conclusion

Injectables are still comparatively unfamiliar in Britain but the studies which have been done over the past ten to fifteen years are encouraging. DMPA has a higher reliability than the progestagen-only Pill but many of the same side effects, especially interference with the menstrual cycle. It is comparatively easy to use, though the need to go back to a doctor or clinic every two or three months can be a drawback. The main problems are that any side effects must be borne until the drug wears off, and that there is a possibility of misuse by some doctors.

The IUD

The IUD, or intra-uterine contraceptive device (more properly called the IUCD), is a device which is inserted into the womb and left there for a considerable time to ensure that no pregnancy can develop. There are actually a large number of IUDs of various shapes and sizes but most of them are about an inch and a half long and rather less than that in width. They are usually made of a type of plastic, and some of them have fine copper wire round a part of them. They usually have a 'tail' of one or two threads which hang into the vagina: this is to make removal easier and enables you to check that the IUD is in place.

The IUD is put into the womb through an applicator. Because the plastic used has a 'memory' the IUD can be flattened out in its applicator, a narrow tube, and as the applicator is removed it will spring into its proper shape. This flexibility allows it to be straightened out easily for removal.

Nobody really knows how an IUD works, but most people think that, like the Pill, it probably has several different ways of preventing pregnancy. One may be that it makes the egg travel faster down the Fallopian tube so that it is still not fully mature when it arrives in the womb, and the womb itself is not ready to receive it. Another theory is that the womb reacts to the presence of a foreign body, so does not distinguish between the IUD and a fertilised egg, and thus stops a fertilised egg from being implanted in its lining. The antibodies created by the reaction to the presence of an IUD may also attack sperm. Because IUDs are effective as soon as they are fitted, it is thought that most of their contraceptive effects must take place within the womb itself, so this means that conception will probably have occurred, but the fertilised egg is prevented from being embedded in the lining of the womb.

New IUDs, which have copper wire on them, or which contain hormones, are probably even more complicated in the variety of ways in which they work.

The IUD does not have any effect on the hormones which

regulate the menstrual cycle, so you go on ovulating and having periods in the usual way.

Background

IUDs were developed in the early years of this century and were made of gold, silver and silk. These early ones were not terribly satisfactory, so IUDs became unpopular until new types of polyethylene were developed and with them a new generation of IUDs.

The reason there are so many different IUD shapes – probably more than a hundred have been described around the world – is that, just as there is no perfect contraceptive, so there is no single ideal IUD. An IUD should be effective in stopping you getting pregnant, easy to fit, and it should stay comfortably in the womb until you want it removed. In fact, though, a device which is small enough to be inserted easily, also falls out more easily, while a large one may stay put but cause discomfort or bleeding.

As a result, there are fashions in IUD design. These fashions may be reflected by the doctor who advises you, but they probably don't matter unless you suffer discomfort with the IUD your doctor selects. In that case, you should ask to try a different type.

Although use of IUDs has grown steadily over the years in Britain, it is still not widespread, compared with the Pill or condom. Around half a million women a year are fitted with an IUD, but most IUD-users have already had a baby. This is partly because the earlier versions, especially, were difficult to use if you had not had a child as they were more difficult to fit. Although the newer IUDs – especially the copper ones – have largely got round this problem, there is a renewal of belief that IUDs may not be suitable for young women who have not yet had any children.

Safety

Whether or not your IUD is inserted safely and without discomfort, and whether or not you are able to wear it easily,

Fitting an IUD

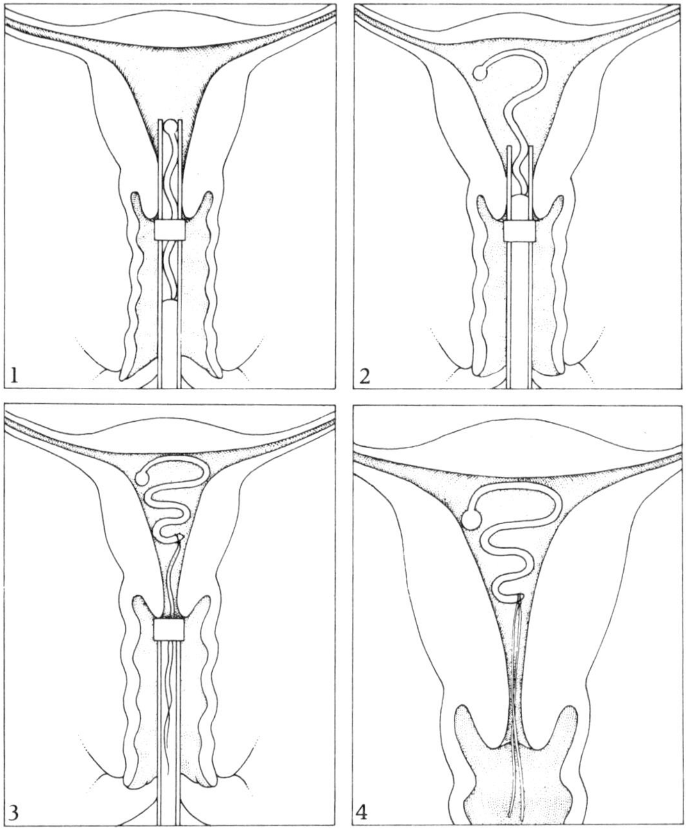

Lippes Loop
1 & 2 A Lippes Loop being introduced by a plunger into the womb and taking on its proper shape
3 & 4 The Lippes in position in the womb with the introducer being withdrawn, leaving the removal threads hanging

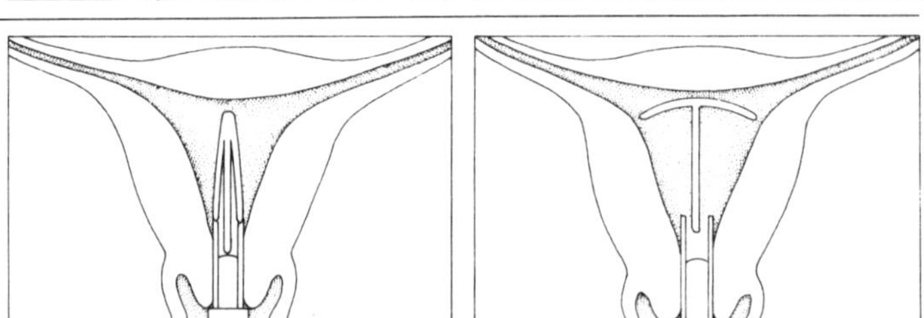

Copper-T
1 The Copper-T being inserted, and **2** the outer tube being withdrawn so that the arms are released

depends as much on who fits it as on the particular device. Putting in an IUD is a skill which improves with practice, and most of the side effects which we describe here are less frequent if the provider of the IUD is somebody who fits them regularly.

Fitting When you have an IUD fitted, a long thin introducer is slid into the womb through the cervical canal. Then, depending on the type, either the IUD may be pushed out of the introducer by a sort of plunger, or the introducer may be put right up to the top of the womb and the device held there by an inner rod while the introducer tube is withdrawn. Once that has been done the rod is taken away leaving the IUD in place. Yet another type consists of a hollow tube in which the device rests.

A few women get very severe cramps when an IUD is fitted. For most, the fitting is virtually painless and it only takes a few minutes, but those most likely to get severe cramps are women without children or those who have not had a child for some years. The cramps seldom last long and can be relieved with mild pain-killing drugs, such as aspirin.

Perforation One rare but serious complication at this stage is that the IUD penetrates the wall of the womb. If this happens, the IUD cannot get lost – it will not work its way round the body, as some people fear. It will lodge in whichever organ or muscle or other part of the body is close to the area of womb where the perforation is. Most of the women who have a perforation simply do not notice it, or have any symptoms, and the perforation is only discovered when they cannot feel the threads or if they become pregnant. It is not unlikely that the reason will be pregnancy, because if the IUD has perforated the wall of the womb, it will not be in the right place to act as a contraceptive.

Sometimes a perforation can lead to an irritation, or a build-up of adhesions around the device, and then it is likely to be noticed – the IUD will have to be removed.

Infection The most serious ill-effect of an IUD otherwise is an increase in your chances of a pelvic infection. If you have undiagnosed gonorrhoea, or gonorrhoea which is not fully treated, when the IUD is inserted, it could flare up again after the fitting. If you have any other sort of vaginal infection, having an IUD fitted can carry it up into the womb. It is very important that you are checked for pelvic infections beforehand and, if necessary, have them cleared up before you use an IUD.

Unfortunately, though, once you have an IUD you do have a slightly higher risk of developing pelvic inflammatory disease than people not using any contraceptive, and a much higher one than people using the Pill or barrier methods, both of which have a protective effect. This remains true for as long as you are wearing an IUD. If you have a number of sexual partners and are under 30, the risk is greater.

It is not clear why there is this increased risk, although one theory is that it may be something to do with the threads attached to the IUD which hang down into the vagina. But because there are different ways in which pelvic inflammatory disease can show itself, and different organisms involved, it may take a long time to work out why this particular side effect should be more common among IUD-users, and how to prevent it.

Pelvic inflammatory disease is usually quite easily treated with antibiotics once it is noticed. Symptoms may include a change to a more irregular or painful menstrual pattern, slight discomfort on intercourse, a vaginal discharge, backache or abdominal pains. You should always see a doctor if you experience any of these problems when using an IUD. If untreated, pelvic inflammatory disease, which includes an inflammation of the Fallopian tubes, may lead to permanent sterility. If the tubes are badly damaged, recurrent attacks of pain, and sexual difficulties, may continue. Very rarely, a neglected infection can result in death.

Bleeding and pain The most common side effects from an IUD are bleeding and pain. When an IUD is first fitted, you will almost certainly have some bleeding for the first couple of days, and during the first two or three months you may experience heavier periods and some irregular bleeding or spotting in between your periods. Some women, though, find that their bodies do not settle down after the first few months, and that they continue to have intermittent spotting and/or very heavy and perhaps painful periods. This may also cause anaemia – though this is less common in Britain than in some countries in the third world, where poor diet and frequent childbearing mean that women are far more susceptible to anaemia.

Pain – either low backache or cramp-like period pains – is also fairly common immediately after an IUD is fitted and perhaps for the first few weeks afterwards as the womb tries to expel the device. A few women continue to feel unacceptable levels of discomfort or pain, and they may need to have the IUD removed.

During the first month, you may also get a vaginal discharge which should disappear after your first period. If it does not, it could be a symptom of vaginal infection or of pelvic inflammatory disease and you should see a doctor.

Expulsion Although you may find it difficult to believe that it can easily fall out, an IUD can do just that. What is more, some women do not notice that it has fallen out.

About half of the IUDs which are going to fall out do so during the first three months, so you need to be particularly careful during that time to check the threads regularly. (The doctor who fits it will show you how to do this.) You need to continue to check the strings during the first year, too, because most of the remaining IUDs which fall out do so during the rest of the first year.

The younger you are, and the fewer children you have had, the more likely you are to have your IUD expelled. Once one has been expelled, the likelihood of your also losing a replacement is increased, even if you are fitted with one of a different shape.

Pregnancy You could get pregnant because the IUD is expelled without your noticing it, or because the wall of the womb has been perforated. More commonly, though, you could get pregnant with the IUD in place, although the rates are quite low (see the section on Effectiveness). If you do get pregnant while wearing an IUD, the pregnancy is more likely to end in a spontaneous abortion. There is also a slightly increased risk, if you leave the IUD there, of a premature birth or bleeding later in pregnancy. Although many women have had their babies perfectly successfully with an IUD still in place, if you do get pregnant it is better, whenever possible, to have the IUD removed.

Another reason for having it removed is that – very rarely but with serious consequences if it happens – a pregnancy may end in a septic abortion during the fourth to sixth month. This was more common with a kind of IUD called the Dalkon Shield, which was withdrawn in 1975. It was recommended then that no new Dalkon Shields should be fitted and that women wearing them should have them replaced with another IUD when they next returned for a check-up. Most of them have been removed by now, but if you are using one still, it should be removed.

Of the pregnancies that occur with an IUD in place, the proportion of ectopic pregnancies is higher than the proportion among women not using contraceptives. An ectopic pregnancy – in which the egg becomes embedded other than in the womb – may produce one-sided abdominal pain followed by bleeding; you should always see a doctor if you have these symptoms while using an IUD, or if you simply suspect you may be pregnant. It is still not clear whether an IUD actually causes more ectopic pregnancies – by interfering with the movement of the fertilised egg, for instance – or whether it is just that IUDs prevent pregnancies within the womb more effectively than they prevent the ones outside it.

There is no evidence that if you get pregnant while using an IUD you are more likely to have a baby born with an abnormality, or to have any special difficulty in getting pregnant when you later want to.

Reasons for not using an IUD

There are a few women for whom an IUD is not a suitable contraceptive. If you have a history of pelvic inflammatory disease, or have had an ectopic pregnancy, or if you have fibroids or a womb which for some other reason is oddly-shaped, or suffer from organic heart disease, you should consider another method. If you have some other gynaecological condition which is being investigated, like unexplained bleeding, or a possible cancer, it is unlikely that a doctor would be willing to give you an IUD until the investigations were complete. If you have an allergy to copper, of course, it would not be wise to use a copper-bearing IUD. You should go back to your family practitioner or clinic at once if you have a vaginal discharge, a late period, abdominal pains or backache or a temperature apparently unconnected with any illness – these could be symptoms of PID or an ectopic pregnancy.

Effectiveness

The skill, speed and confidence of the person who fits your IUD is very important in determining how well it works. Failure rates vary quite a bit from country to country and they also vary from place to place within a country and even within the same clinic, depending on the particular doctor or nurse. On the whole, there is a failure rate of something over two for every hundred women in each year. An IUD is effective from the time it is fitted. Once it is inserted, however, the failure rate isn't influenced so much by you as with most other methods – you can't forget to use it or take a risk – but you will need to check the strings carefully, especially during the first year, to make sure the IUD has not fallen out.

There are no problems over long-term storage and deterioration. An IUD should be sterile when it is fitted, and in Britain they are usually supplied in sterile disposable packs. If they are not, they will be sterilised immediately before being inserted.

At one time it was not clear whether IUDs would continue

to work over a long period of time, and you were usually told to have your IUD removed and replaced every two years. Now it is known that the ordinary plastic ones can be left in the womb for much longer than that and if there are no problems you may be able to keep yours for some years. The practice is different for the copper-bearing IUDs, which are newer. It is known that the copper gradually wears off, but it is less certain how important that is in continuing to prevent pregnancy. The manufacturers therefore recommend that copper-bearing IUDs are removed after two or three years (depending on the type).

Because so much depends on an IUD being large enough to stay in place, but not too big to be uncomfortable, it has been suggested that IUDs would work better if they were custom-fitted for every woman. Tests are going on in Britain to find ways to measure the exact size and shape of your womb, so that an IUD can be chosen to match it, and to see if this will result in fewer side effects and more reliable protection against pregnancy. Although early results are encouraging, it is not yet clear that they are good enough to justify the enormous extra effort and expense involved.

Acceptability

An IUD is a pretty reliable method of contraception, one which is easy to use, requires only the minimum of attention once it is in place, and is discreet. You don't have to think about it at all except to check the threads, though this checking may be a problem among women who have a cultural or personal dislike of placing their fingers in their vagina.

You will probably have to be prepared to have full medical examination before the IUD is inserted, as the doctor or clinic will need to know various things about you in order to make sure you are likely to be suited to an IUD.

Unless you suffer from intermittent bleeding or cramps – and these are the most common reasons women give for abandoning an IUD – you and your partner have almost no reason even to know an IUD is there. A few men do notice the strings, and some complain that they are slightly scratched by them – if this happens, the strings have probably been trimmed to the wrong length. They can easily be tidied up if you go back to the person who fitted the IUD. It could, however, be an indication that your IUD is slipping out, especially if the effect is suddenly noticeable after you have worn the IUD for a while. In any event, you should have it checked.

The increased chances of pelvic inflammatory disease (PID) are what concern many IUD-users, particularly if they have not yet had children. To put this risk into perspective, you need to look at it against the risk in the population generally, as well as against the risk of it occurring if you are using other contraceptives. Barrier methods and the Pill have a protective effect against PID, though of course they have their own disadvantages. The risk to an IUD-user is not much greater than that found in the population as a whole, unless you are young and have a variety of partners – or may have. Or unless you have a Casanova as a boyfriend.

If you are in a stable sexual relationship the IUD may be a good choice, but it is probably less of a good bet if you are in your teens or early twenties with no immediate intention of settling with one man. Apart from the question of PID, there is a higher expulsion rate among users who have not had a child, even with the newer IUDs. On the other hand, because IUDs are so easy to use, and don't need any action at the time of sexual activity, they could be very useful if you have a rather erratic sex life and do not want to keep taking the Pill. One possible way of reducing the risks is to use a spermicide in addition to an IUD. This will reduce still further the failure rate, and your chances of PID, without demanding too much extra effort. Alternatively, you could use a sheath as a precaution.

If you have always had painful or very heavy periods, an IUD is likely to make things worse, rather than better, and so may not be a suitable answer for your contraceptive requirements.

Availability

An IUD is normally fitted by a doctor. There are a small number of specially trained nurses who fit IUDs, but they are rare. In fact, there is evidence from many countries that the person who fits an IUD does not necessarily have to be a medically trained doctor as such, and in many countries you find not only nurses but people like health auxiliaries putting in IUDs – with results which are as good as those of the doctors. What is important is that the person who fits an IUD is specially trained to do it, and does it regularly. Like any skill, it is better if it is practised often.

So while you can only get an IUD from your doctor or a family planning clinic, if you are going to your GP there are some questions you need to ask. Many family practitioners have now undertaken special IUD training courses, and may be excellent inserters. Because they may know you well, they may have a good relationship with you which makes the fitting easier and more relaxed. If they do a number of IUD insertions – two or three a week, for example – they will also have the practice which makes the fitting quicker and safer. If these conditions do not apply, you may find it preferable, for this particular method of contraception, to go to a family planning clinic.

At a family planning clinic you will see a doctor or nurse who is specially trained in IUD insertions. Whoever it is will be doing a large number of insertions regularly, and should be used to discussing all the aspects of IUD use in detail. Most will be understanding and sympathetic about possible pain, or your nervousness – though this is not invariably true, as familiarity can breed a certain impatience. Finally, a clinic doctor or nurse is more likely to be a woman – and you can certainly ask to see a woman doctor when making your appointment.

Clinics are generally less conveniently located than your local doctor's surgery; with an IUD you are likely to be asked to come back for a follow-up visit after three months, and then at yearly intervals only.

Whether you choose to go to your own doctor or a clinic, you may be asked to make an appointment during the time of your next period, or in the first few days after it. This is because IUDs are easier to fit then, because of changes in the cervix which make it simpler to slide the inserter through. It also ensures that you are unlikely to be pregnant when the IUD is fitted. This can be a nuisance if you have just had a period and are going to have to wait nearly a month before getting your IUD, as you will have to use another method meanwhile. An IUD can be fitted at any time during your cycle, though, and if you think it is really urgent to have one fitted straight away, you can probably get this arranged.

Like most methods of contraception, the fitting of most IUDs is free under the National Health Service, and so is the cost of the devices in common use. However the cost to the NHS of the different devices varies considerably, so your doctor or clinic may be unwilling to prescribe a particular type unless there is a good medical reason.

If your own GP is reluctant to fit you with an IUD but you prefer the thought of a family doctor doing it rather than a clinic, or if there is no clinic near you, you can get the list of other doctors who will provide contraception for people other than their own registered patients from any post office or from your local Family Practitioner Committee. The FPC might also be able to tell you which of those doctors have been trained in IUD insertions, or offer an IUD service.

Types of IUD

Although there is a wide variety of IUD designs, there are currently several which are popular in Britain, and which are on the FPA's recommended list. They are in two groups, the plain plastic ones and the copper-wire-bearing ones.

Plastic devices The Lippes Loop (made by Ortho) is considered suitable mainly for women who have had at least one child. It is probably the oldest established of the traditional IUDs and has been used successfully for a number of years. The Lippes Loop is a snaking zigzag which widens at the top with a double thread attached, for ease of removal and so

Types of IUD

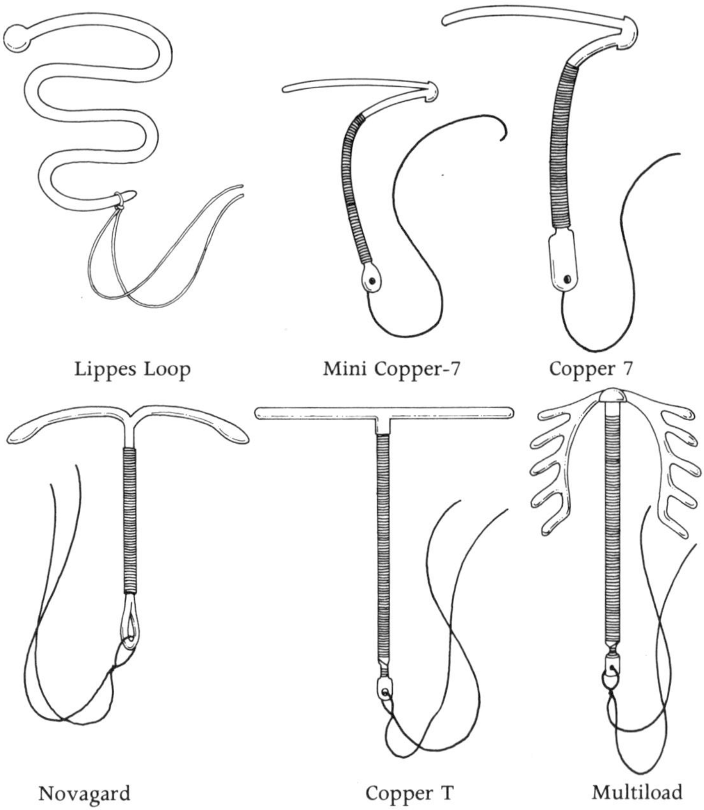

that you can check the IUD is still in place. Another popular device, the Saf-T-Coil, is no longer manufactured but if you've got one there's no need to have it replaced.

Copper-bearing IUDs The Copper-7 and the Copper-T (made by G.D. Searle and Ortho) are considered suitable for childless women as well as those with children, mainly because of ease of insertion. A new smaller version of the Copper 7 is now available and awaiting approval by the FPA. Another copper-bearing IUD, the Multiload Cu250, made by Organon, provides a high-protection rate against pregnancy with a low expulsion and removal rate, but this is generally confined to women who have had a baby. All three devices have a length of fine copper wire wound round their stems which in some way helps to ensure that the womb rejects, or is made unwelcoming for, a fertilised egg. A further copper-bearing IUD – the Novagard (manufactured by G.D. Searle) – has a silver core. Because of the intensified effect of these four devices, a smaller-sized IUD can be fitted which reduces the side effects of cramp and bleeding, and may reduce the chances of expulsion as well.

Other IUDs Some IUDs contain a hormone which can be released steadily into the womb and have a more local effect than swallowing the Pill. They are not generally available in Britain yet and are described in the chapter on New Horizons.

Conclusion

An IUD is probably the easiest and most convenient method of contraception – if you are able to use it and don't have more than one sexual partner (or can trust your sexual partners). But although the number of serious ill-effects is not large, those which cause discomfort or bleeding are common enough to make a proportion of those women who try an IUD give it up subsequently.

It is still less well accepted by young women or those who have not had children both because they are more likely to suffer side effects, or expel the IUD, and because of the increased possibility of pelvic inflammatory disease. This is a pity because in many ways it is a particularly good method for people with an irregular sex life – you don't have to worry about a contraceptive at the time of sex, or remember to keep taking something whether or not you are sexually active at any given time.

Periodic abstinence

The methods used in periodic abstinence are all based on the supposition that if you can determine when an egg is released from its follicle, and avoid having sex around that time, you can also avoid getting pregnant. There are various ways of trying to determine when the egg is released, either based on the timing of your menstrual cycle – the rhythm, or calendar, method – or on changes which take place in the body at around the time of ovulation – the temperature method, and the ovulation method (sometimes called the Billings method).

During the first part of the cycle, there is no egg around to be fertilised. At mid-cycle, the luteinising hormone LH is released from the pituitary and triggers off the bursting of a follicle to release an egg. The egg travels down the Fallopian tube to arrive in the womb and, unless it is fertilised, it can only survive for a day or less in the tube.

At the time of ovulation, a number of other changes begin to take place in the body. Your temperature rises slightly; many of the chemicals in your body alter; and the mucus in your cervix increases in amount and becomes more watery, to help the sperm on their way to the egg. Your urine and sweat contain more oestrogens, too.

Between 12 and 16 days after ovulation, menstrual bleeding takes place, and the cycle begins again.

Because menstruation always takes place from 12 to 16 days after ovulation, it is very easy to calculate backwards and discover when you ovulated. If you have a regular cycle, and have kept accurate records over a year, you will be able to work out a pattern of the days when you are most likely to be fertile.

Unfortunately, it is much more difficult to predict in advance, from the beginning of the cycle, the day you will ovulate. This is important because while the egg only lives for up to 24 hours, sperm are now known to be able to live for three days and possibly longer. So avoiding intercourse once you have ovulated is not enough – you must add at least three days beforehand to the time during which you don't have sex. Because the changes in your body become most evident at the time of ovulation, you can use them as a marker but not as a predictor.

The Calendar method

This is often called the 'rhythm method' or, more unkindly, 'Vatican Roulette'.

The first day of your cycle is the day that your menstrual bleeding begins. The egg will be released between 12 and 16 days before the next menstrual period, which gives a minimum of five days which are 'unsafe'. You must add an extra day to those to cover the time during which an egg might survive, and add on another four days at the beginning to cover the time a sperm might live. That gives you a total of ten 'unsafe' days. So if you have an absolutely regular cycle of 28 days, the calculation would look like this:

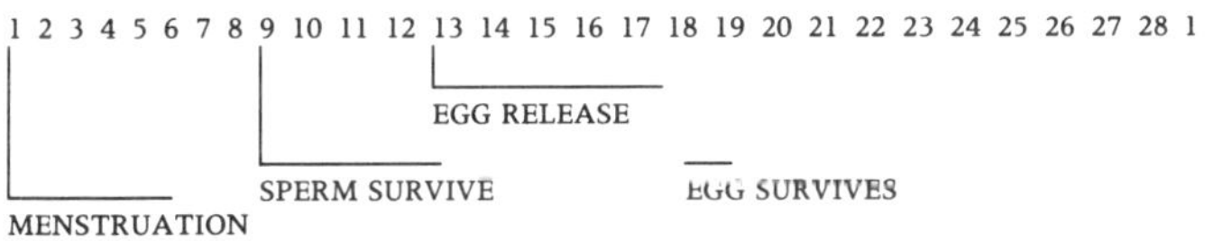

Very few women have a cycle which is that exact, so the calculations for most of them get more complicated. You have to allow for the variations in your cycle by keeping a record of the number of days in the cycle (worked out from the date of the start of each period) for at least eight cycles, and preferably 12. You will then know the longest and shortest cycles you are likely to have (at least in normal circumstances, because all sorts of things from illness to air travel can affect your cycle). Several formulae for doing the calculation have been worked out, but this is a generally agreed one.

In your shortest cycle you will probably have ovulated earliest – subtract 18 days from the number of days in that cycle. This will give you your first 'unsafe' day.

Then take the number of days in your longest cycle, and

subtract 11; this gives you the last 'unsafe' day. You should avoid intercourse in any cycle between those two days.

The diagram shows how this would work out for somebody whose cycles varied between 26 and 30 days. Her first possible fertile day would be 26–18, or day 8 – the eighth day after bleeding starts. Her last possible day would be 30–11, or day 19. The 'safe' days during which she could have sex would be during the first week of her cycle and then on or after day 20 of her cycle. She would have to assume that she was fertile for 12 days of her cycle, and avoid sex during that period.

There are various mechanical calculators available for working out this formula, but they do nothing to improve its accuracy. They depend on your having kept exact records of your cycles and then they simply do the same calculation we have done here. They might be useful for the non-mathematically-minded as a check on the sums.

The calendar method, used alone, is the least reliable version of periodic abstinence.

Temperature method

During or just after ovulation, a woman's basal body temperature will rise by about half a degree and stay up for some days. The rise happens over about a forty-eight hour period. Allowing another twenty-four hours to be absolutely certain that the egg has not survived in the tubes, you can then assume that you are no longer fertile.

If you then use the calendar method and a temperature chart, you calculate the first 'unsafe' day from the calendar in the way explained, but you work out the last 'unsafe' day as three days after your temperature has reached a plateau at its higher level. This is somewhat more reliable than using the calendar method on its own.

For greater reliability, avoid sex altogether from the first day of your cycle until three days after your temperature has reached a plateau at its higher level.

A rise in temperature of half a degree is quite small, so it needs to be measured with accuracy. Take your temperature

The temperature method

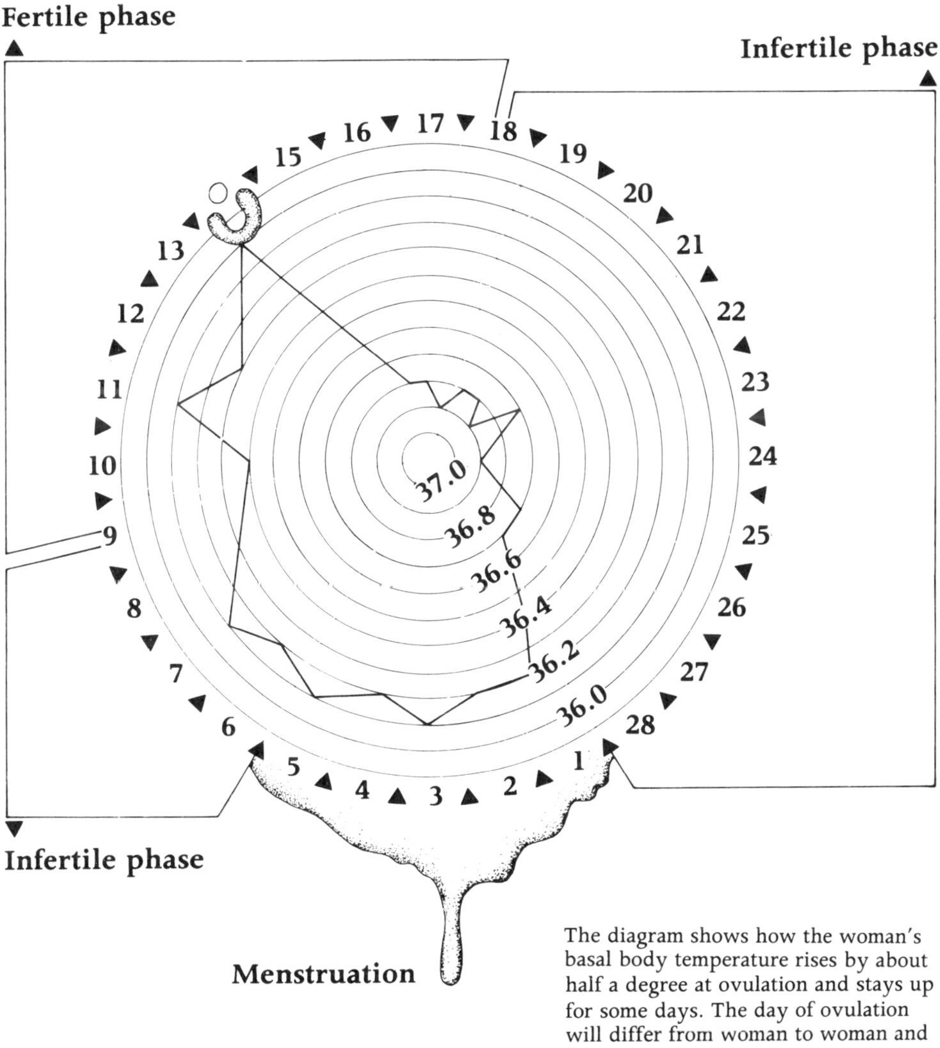

The diagram shows how the woman's basal body temperature rises by about half a degree at ovulation and stays up for some days. The day of ovulation will differ from woman to woman and from cycle to cycle.

by mouth first thing in the morning, before getting out of bed and before taking any hot food or drink. (Mothers of young babies may find it difficult to take their temperatures consistently after a period of rest.) If you use an ordinary clinical thermometer you must keep it under your tongue for a good four minutes, regardless of what the manufacturer's instructions say.

To record your temperature, you can either make yourself a simple chart using graph paper, or you can buy a ready-made temperature chart. These are available from some chemists', or by mail order from Family Planning Sales Limited. A year's supply should cost around £1.20. Family planning clinics and the Catholic Marriage Advisory Council also have charts and will help you to understand and use the system.

Cervical mucus method

This is sometimes described as the 'Billings method' or the 'Peak symptom' method. The mucus which is secreted in the cervix and lies in the vagina varies quite a lot during the month. During the first days after bleeding, there is almost no mucus but gradually more discharge begins to appear. At this time it is normally whiteish, cloudy and sticky. Around the time of ovulation, the mucus changes and becomes clear and much more slippery, as well as runnier. This mucus can be felt at the vulva, which will feel wet and slippery. The transparent runny mucus only lasts for a few days and then changes back to the whiteish, cloudy and thicker sort.

If you avoid sex from the time that the whiteish discharge begins early in the cycle, to the time when it reappears after the thin runny sort, you will probably have avoided the peak fertile period. You can be shown how to recognise the different stages of the mucus, either by smearing some on to a chemically treated paper rather like litmus paper, which will change colour as the consistency of the mucus changes, or simply by its look and feel. In Britain, the chemical paper is not used, as it is considered less reliable than learning to recognise the changes as they apply to you.

Sympto-thermal method

Many people combine the temperature method and the mucus method in order to try and get a cross-check on the symptoms which will help to indicate the time of ovulation.

The most reliable study comparing the cervical mucus method with the sympto-thermal method suggested very little difference in pregnancy rates, which were around 20–24 per hundred women in a year.

Background

There has been a long history of attempts to develop a 'safe period', but for a long time, because the menstrual cycle was not clearly understood, it was thought that the peak period of fertility was at the beginning of the menstrual cycle. It was only in the 1930s that the calendar (rhythm) method as it is known today was developed.

An enormous amount of research is going on into the method in an effort to make it more reliable. This is partly because if you could ensure its reliability, you could cut down the amount of time that at present you have to avoid sex during each cycle, which would make it more acceptable. If this worked, then there would undoubtedly be a lot of couples who would prefer it to the more cumbersome barriers, or to the Pill and IUD with their more serious ill-effects. A 'safe period' is the only method of family planning that the Vatican accepts. Some of the research ideas which could improve the method are outlined under 'New Horizons'.

Safety

Side effects from using the safe period seem to be few, as you might expect. The most serious possibility is that, if you do get pregnant, it could have an effect on the pregnancy itself or on the baby (see below).

Congenital effects There is evidence from animal studies and one human study that using old sperm (that was ejaculated a few days before fertilisation) can increase the chances of congenital abnormalities in the offspring. In

Cervical mucus method

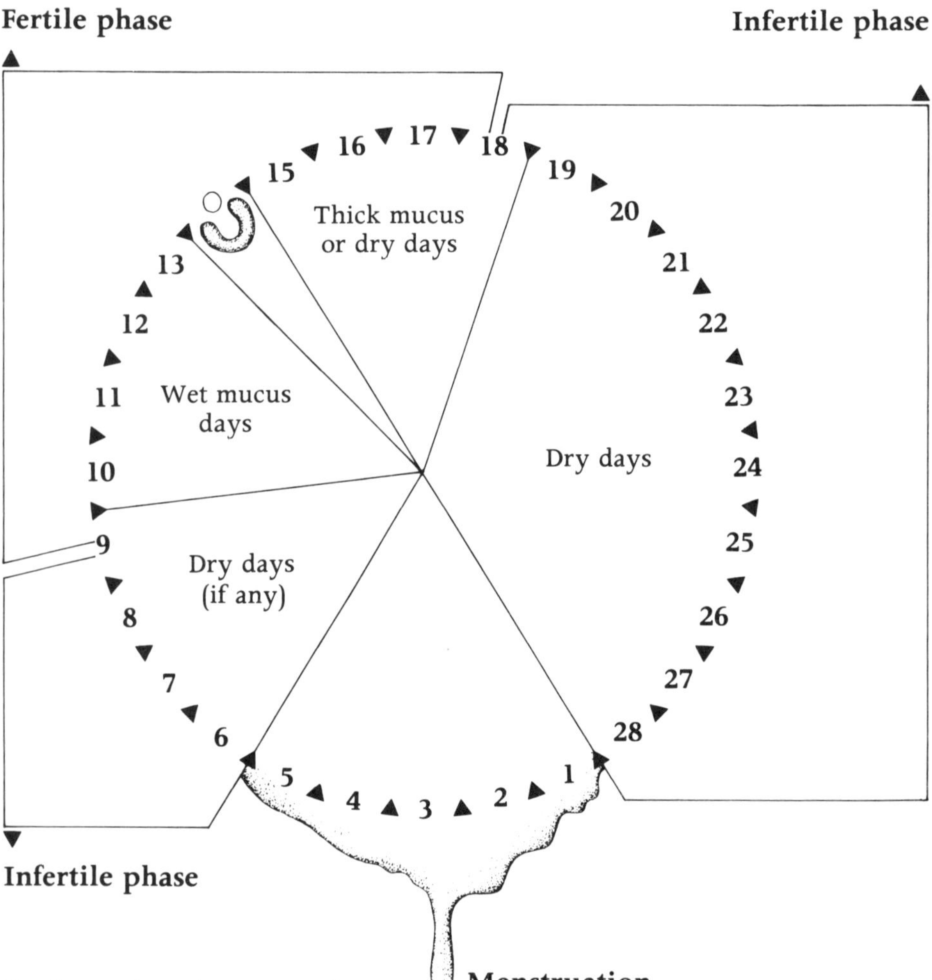

The diagram shows the sequence of dry and wet mucus days around the time of ovulation, and indicates the fertile and infertile phases.

theory, if you do get pregnant while using the safe period, fertilisation would have been more likely to have involved some ageing sperm. For instance, if you ovulate earlier than you expect to, some of the sperm from an act of sex three days before may still be alive and able to fertilise the egg. However, there is no clear evidence among humans that this is a real danger. (It would be difficult to prove because many users of the 'safe period' are Catholics who may have a different genetic background to the rest of the population, or have a different diet or other environmental factors.) The possibility of congenital abnormalities remains a possibility, but no more.

Abnormal pregnancy There is also a little evidence to suggest that if the egg is fertilised late in the menstrual cycle, the chances of that pregnancy being ectopic could be increased, as could be the chances of placenta praevia. Again, this is a possibility but not more.

Effectiveness

Cyclical methods depend, like most other methods of contraception, on careful use, with the additional snag that they demand quite long periods of abstinence. As a result, how well they work depends very much on your enthusiasm and determination, and good results in one study have often been balanced by poor ones in another.

But it can be said that the calendar method on its own is the least effective, and that a combination of methods tends to work better than any of them alone. If you use both the mucus and temperature method, there is probably a pregnancy rate of something about 20 per hundred woman-years. Some very enthusiastic users claim much better results.

If you have very uneven menstrual cycles, with a difference of more than ten days between the longest and the shortest, you will either find that the 'safe' period is tiny or even non-existent, or you will have to take risks which will increase the chances of pregnancy.

Working out the safe period – an example

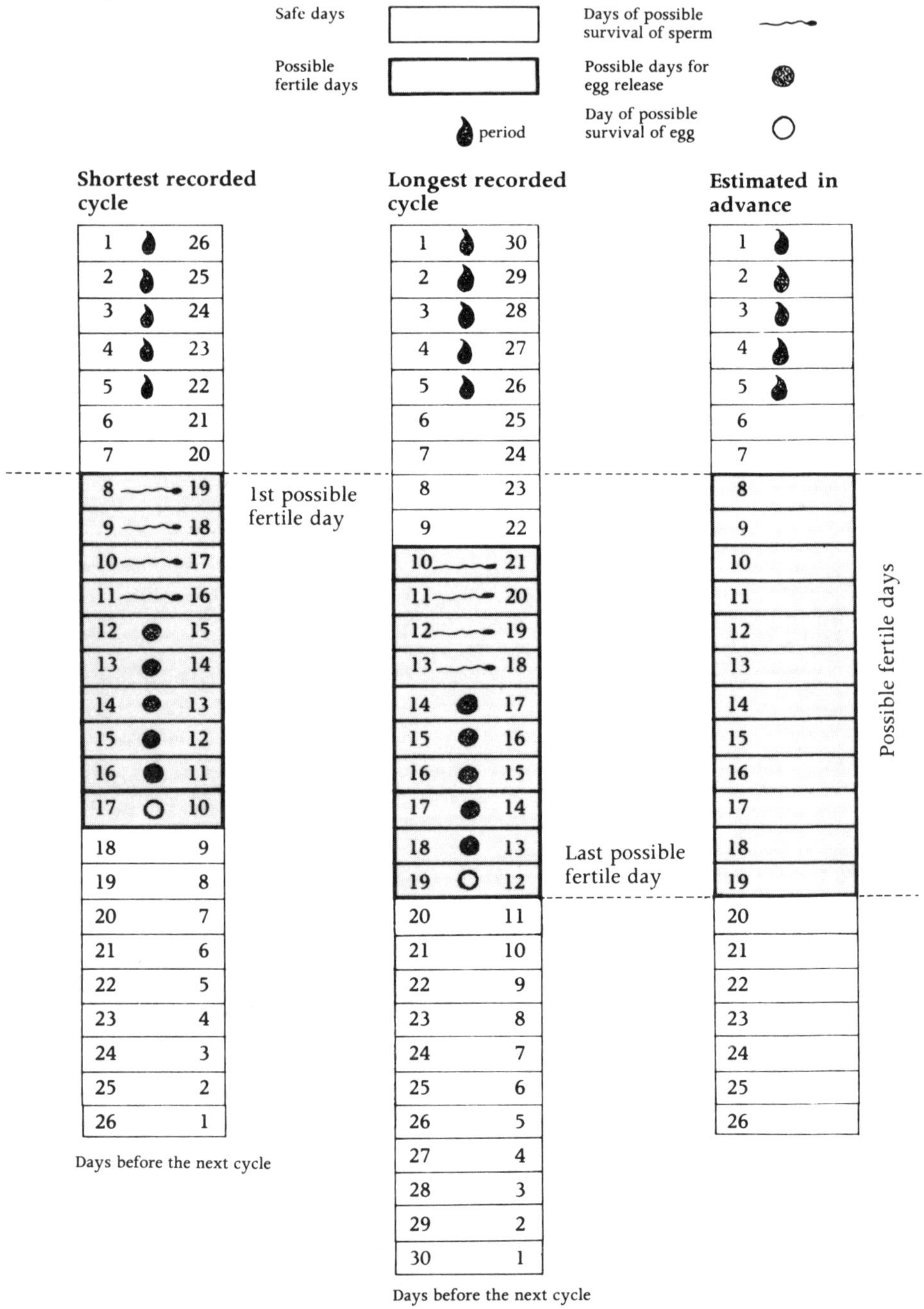

However regular your cycle normally is, it can be affected by all sorts of things. A recent abortion or pregnancy will alter it and you should not rely on rhythm for four months after the abortion or birth of the child. A sudden physical or emotional upset will also affect your cycle. So may any illness – even if it does not cause a rise in temperature which will make your temperature chart useless – or a sudden strenuous effort, or travel. You should avoid relying on the 'safe' period at such times.

Acceptability

Although this is the only method accepted by the Catholic Church, various surveys suggest that in Britain most Catholics use the same spread of contraceptive methods as the rest of the population. Nevertheless, for those who do follow the Catholic Church's ruling, there is not much question of acceptability – it is the 'safe period' or nothing.

But there has been renewed interest in cyclical methods recently among women's groups and those looking for a more 'natural' lifestyle. For them the lack of side effects or of interference with the body's natural systems is a great plus, and one for which they will be prepared to sacrifice some reliability. If you feel like this you are likely in any case to be an enthusiastic and meticulous user of the method, which will reduce the chances of failure.

You may also feel that the mucus method helps you to understand and get accustomed to your own body. On the other hand, if you dislike handling your vulva, the mucus method is not likely to be suitable.

Periodic abstinence is probably less well suited to those with a varied sex life or an intermittent one. Admittedly there is no need for advance preparation, or for last-minute fumbling, but the fact that you have entered the first 'unsafe' day of your cycle does not mesh well with casual sex. Nor is it very appealing if, for example, your partner is working on a North Sea oil rig and only comes home on what may turn out to be the wrong days of the month.

Some couples find the restriction of sex to certain days can itself be rather inhibiting, or just plain frustrating. Others say that the sense of shared concern brought about by such a discipline actually helps towards a tender and loving relationship.

Periodic abstinence may be more acceptable to older women, whose fertility is decreasing – though the costs of failure of the method may be higher for them, as the incidence of abnormal babies, and of other hazards associated with pregnancy, rises sharply once you are over 35. In the pre-menopausal years, however, as in the teens, ovulation may be erratic making the method difficult to use.

Some people reduce the possibilities of pregnancy with these methods by combining them with a barrier or another form of contraception. They may, for example, use a condom during the 'unsafe' days and nothing during the 'safe' period. Many use the method in combination with coitus interruptus so that they avoid using a mechanical contraceptive at all – though this is not approved by the Catholic Church, all the same. Combining barrier and cyclical methods of contraception does reduce your chances of pregnancy, and cut down the number of occasions on which you have to use a barrier, which can be an advantage if you don't much like them.

One major drawback of the calendar method, or of the calendar used together with the temperature method, is that you need to go through a large number of cycles before being able to establish what your fertile periods are. To a lesser extent, this applies to all the techniques in this section, as it takes time to recognise with certainty both your temperature pattern and the fluctuations of your cervical mucus. You must either rely on another method while learning, or be extremely vulnerable to pregnancy. If you do get pregnant, of course, it will also interrupt your learning – the cycles will no longer occur. Some people find that the daily temperature-taking, and the need to keep checking the cervical mucus, are a nuisance.

Availability

Although your family planning practitioner or clinic can probably explain the temperature method to you and give general advice on these methods, few have a really detailed knowledge of them. The Catholic National Marriage Guidance Council has a special 'Natural Methods Unit' and will send you the names of teachers of the techniques, especially of the mucus method. So too will the Birmingham Natural Family Planning Unit (see Appendix 3). They have teachers throughout the country who are willing to help.

Conclusion

The types of periodic abstinence are largely harmless and, once you have been taught to use the different techniques, easy to use. They are, however, among the least reliable of contraceptive techniques and to get the best from them you have to be extremely keen to use them and diligent about doing so. The calendar method on its own has the worst failure rate and is not recommended. The temperature and mucus methods both help to pinpoint ovulation more accurately and so shorten the 'unsafe' period, but the temperature method on its own works best if you restrict sex to the second half of the cycle. A combination of temperature and mucus methods has the greatest reliability, though it means that you have to take your temperature each day and feel your cervical mucus for a large part of each cycle.

A major problem with these methods is the erratic nature of most people's cycles, and the unreliability of even the most normally regular cycles if you are ill, upset, on holiday or tired. Another may be the difficulty of confining sex to the 'safe' days. As a result, while it may be enriching for some stable couples, periodic abstinence is not well suited to those whose sex life is intermittent or more casual.

Post-coital contraception

Post-coital contraception is the name given to a whole range of methods, or potential methods, which can be used within hours of an unprotected act of sex, to ensure that you don't get pregnant. None of them is recommended as a routine contraceptive taken after each sex act. The two techniques which are available in Britain should, therefore, be regarded as emergency measures only.

The kinds of emergency as a result of which women ask for post-coital contraception include, besides rape, unexpected sex (particularly very young women having their first sexual experience), or sex when the usual contraception has been forgotten, or is suspected of having failed.

Oestrogens and Progestagens

If you take two tablets of a fairly high-dose combined Pill as soon as possible after unprotected sex, followed by two more tablets after 12 hours, you will be unlikely to get pregnant. This is not a particularly large dose: the two Pills together only amount to the kind of dose taken regularly by Pill-users in the 1960s. As you will see from the section on the Pill, it works in a variety of ways to prevent pregnancy, and it is still not entirely clear which of its various effects can also make it work post-coitally – but it does work.

Background

Research has been carried out to see if oestrogen or progestagen alone would be suitable for post-coital contraception. High doses of oestrogen on its own have been found to prevent pregnancy, but the dose has to be much higher than with a combined Pill and the side-effects – nausea, vomiting, bleeding and breast tenderness – are much worse. Besides, oestrogen is the hormone which produces most of the effects on the circulatory system, so that there may be a risk of thrombosis from these very high doses.

Progestagens used alone can also prevent pregnancy, and in some part of the world they are being used (taken after each act of sex) as a regular method of contraception. There is a fairly high failure rate, though – around 2–4 per 100 woman-years – and the risk goes up if the dose is taken more than three hours after sex.

The idea of using a combined Pill post-coitally is to cut down the risks and side effects of the earlier prototypes with one or other hormone, by reducing the oestrogen dose, and increasing the effectiveness.

Safety

As we said, a comparatively high-dose combined Pill was taken by millions of women during the 1960s. Only a tiny number suffered any serious ill-effects, but even so the dose was later diminished to reduce the risks. It was not a good idea to take these high doses regularly, but there are no serious health risks from a one-off regimen of four tablets over a 12-hour period.

Some women may feel rather sick, and a few vomit. Others may have some irregular bleeding, a headache or breast tenderness. These are only temporary symptoms and will go away within a couple of days.

Effectiveness

Post-coital Pills are very effective if they are taken quickly enough. That means you should start the treatment within 24 hours of sex, if possible, and at the very latest within 72 hours. If the gap between having sex and going for post-coital contraception has been longer than that, there is no point in pretending it hasn't and hoping that the post-coital Pill will nevertheless work. It won't. Nor will it bring about an abortion if a fertilised egg has been successfully implanted in the womb.

Acceptability

As an emergency measure, the post-coital Pill has several advantages. An egg may or may not have been fertilised – you won't know either way. So for women who don't like the thought of aborting an implanted egg, this could be more acceptable.

The other attraction is that if in fact you would have got pregnant it avoids the pregnancy and the need to make a choice between an abortion or continuing with that pregnancy. Getting an abortion, if you did need one, is itself not easy; getting post-coital contraception is very much easier and avoids any kind of clinical procedure.

As a routine method of contraception, the post-coital Pill would be unlikely to be very acceptable, because you would not want to take higher doses of combined oestrogen and progestagen on a regular basis when you can get full contraceptive cover on an ordinary combined Pill with lower health risks.

Availability

The Pill is a drug available on prescription only, so you will have to go to your doctor or a clinic to get post-coital Pills. If your family practitioner provides this service, it will be free under the NHS. If he does not, you will not have time to start looking for another GP who might provide the service, and should get to a clinic quickly. Not all family planning clinics provide a post-coital service, but some do; it is worth a phone call to your local one. Otherwise you will have to go to the Brook Centres, your nearest British Pregnancy Advisory Service centre, the Pregnancy Advisory Service in London or the Marie Stopes Clinic (see page 144). These are not covered by the NHS and you will have to pay around £15 for a post-coital service. As time goes by, more family doctors and clinics are providing post-coital birth control.

Post-coital IUD insertion

If a copper-bearing IUD is inserted within five days of unprotected sex, it too will work as a post-coital contraceptive. There is even more doubt about how an IUD works than there is about the Pill, so it is also unclear why it works post-coitally. But we do know that it is effective as soon as it is put in and that it probably has a variety of effects within the womb itself.

Safety

There is the same possibility of the same side effects that always exist with an IUD (see the section on IUDs for more information).

If it has been more than five days since you had unprotected sex, there is no point in pretending that it hasn't, and having an IUD fitted. It will not cause an abortion if a fertilised egg has become embedded in the womb. Assuming that it is fitted within five days, it should be effective in preventing pregnancy.

Availability

An IUD can be fitted free on the NHS, and involves going to a doctor or clinic. If you want one inserted as a post-coital contraceptive, the important thing is time. You will need to find out whether a local clinic will be able to give you an appointment within five days of the unprotected sex. If your GP fits IUDs you will again need an urgent appointment. If you cannot get an IUD fitted quickly by your GP or local family planning clinic, you will need to find one of the charitable or private organisations which offer a post coital service: the Brook Centres, your nearest British Pregnancy Advisory Service centre, the Pregnancy Advisory Service in London or the Marie Stopes Clinic (see page 144). The cost for a post-coital service at any of these will be around £15. Most charities will only fit an IUD within 72 hours of unprotected sex.

Acceptability

An IUD as a post-coital contraceptive has some of the same advantages as a post-coital Pill. The egg may or may not have been fertilised – you won't know either way, so for women who don't like the thought of aborting, post-coital contraception avoids the moral dilemmas of abortion. And if you would have got pregnant, it avoids the need for an abortion, or for continuing an unwanted pregnancy. As you do not have to get two doctors to agree, it is easier to get than an abortion. For some women, another advantage is that you are fitted with a long-term contraceptive at the same time as getting emergency protection.

For others, that may be a disadvantage of a post-coital IUD, compared to the post-coital Pill. Once you have taken your four Pills, you have finished with the method, and can then make your own choice about which contraceptive to use in future. If you have a post-coital IUD, you are stuck with it until you go back to have it out. (This is a disadvantage which seems to loom larger before you have one inserted than afterwards. Many women who have only reluctantly accepted a post-coital IUD discover, to their own surprise, that they are quite happy with it, and decide to keep it as a contraceptive.) So you can't look at a post-coital IUD simply as a short-term method: you should read the section on IUDs together with this one and decide whether or not an IUD is a good choice for you.

For a few women, it may be the only option. If you suffer from any of the conditions which would make you unsuitable for ordinary combined Pill use, you will probably not be able to get the post-coital Pill either. The IUD may also be the best alternative if it is more than 24 hours since you had unprotected sex, though used post-coitally it may not be a good idea if you think that the sex act could have left you at risk from a sexually transmitted disease.

What you do next

Whether you use the Pill or the IUD for post-coital contraception, you will probably be asked to go back a month later. It is important that you do this to make absolutely sure that you have not got pregnant. If you are pregnant, there is no reason to fear that the baby will have been affected if you used a post-coital Pill, or had an IUD fitted – but you will be offered help with an abortion if you wish. If you decide to keep the baby, it is probably better to have the IUD removed.

Sterilisation

Sterilisation has been done for generations, but in the past it tended to be the last desperate resort of couples who had large families or where the health of the woman was threatened by a further birth. As contraception has become more reliable and more widespread, the trend has changed. Women now have smaller families and have finished having them much earlier.

As more has become known about the possible side effects of the various contraceptives, and particularly about the increased risk to older Pill-users, more and more women have decided that there is little point in continuing reversible contraceptives for the rest of their fertile lives. Over a third of couples over 30 but below their middle-40s have chosen either male or female sterilisation. With every survey, the proportion grows and the age at which people choose sterilisation drops. This is one of the biggest changes in contraceptive habits since the last *Which?* Guide was published.

Male sterilisation

Male sterilisation is called vasectomy. It is a simple operation which involves blocking off the vas deferens so that the sperm are unable to reach the exit through the penis. Sperm go on being made, and travel along the vas as far as they can, but after a while they dissolve and are absorbed into the system. The operation does not involve removing the testicles, and it does not physically affect your sex drive or make you impotent. When you have sex you will ejaculate in the usual way, because the blockage does not affect the seminal fluid which is made near where the vas joins the urethra. The sole difference (visible only under a microscope) is that the seminal fluid won't have sperm in it.

The operation is normally done under a local anaesthetic, though some doctors will use a general anaesthetic. Your pubic hairs may be shaved, and the surgeon will usually make two tiny cuts in the scrotum (one each side, because you have two tubes, one going into each testicle). He then pulls the vas until a loop is visible, ties it in two places and

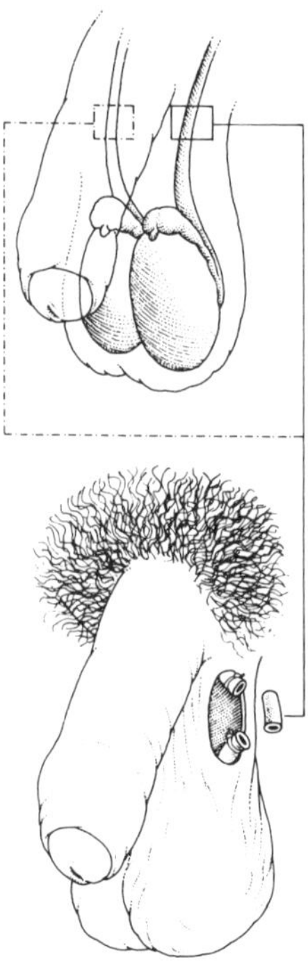

cuts out the short length in between. You have about 45 cm of vas deferens, so pulling out a small loop is less alarming than it sounds, but you will probably feel some discomfort at the back of the abdomen. The whole operation only lasts a few minutes, and you may not even need a stitch in the scrotum if the cut is small.

After the operation, you are likely to feel discomfort for a couple of days or up to a week, and possibly see some bruising of the skin. You will be advised to wear a scrotal support or tight-fitting under-pants during that time – you should take some with you when you go for the operation, too. You should avoid doing anything too strenuous, like lifting heavy weights, for a couple of days.

There have been claims, by a few men, that they have had sex within an hour or so of the operation. Most, however, are too sore for the first few days to enjoy it. Regardless of when you resume sexual activity, though, other contraceptive methods must be used until the sperm count is clear.

If you think you might want a vasectomy you should be absolutely certain that you will not want any more children. Although some doctors have had quite good results from rejoining the two ends of the vas, you could never be sure that you would be able to fertilise an egg even if the join was successful. A ring of scar tissue often grows around the join and prevents the sperm getting through. You should assume that the result is permanent.

There have been attempts to design a plug to fit in the vas to make reversibility easier – either the plug could be removed, or it could have a kind of valve or tap in it (nicknamed a 'stop-cock') so that when you wanted to produce a baby the tap could be turned on. To date none of these efforts has been very successful – partly because of scar tissue growing around the plug and blocking the vas even more effectively, and partly because a high proportion of men who have undergone a vasectomy operation develop antibodies to sperm (there is more about antibodies under Safety.)

Safety

Vasectomy is a very safe procedure. The most common short-term problems with it are bleeding after the operation, or an infection. Bleeding may just lead to your being told to rest at home, but if a large area of internal bleeding builds up you might have to go into hospital to have it drained to avoid infection. If you do get a swelling in the scrotum, you should go and see your doctor immediately. Very rarely there are other long-term complications, like a secondary infection, a fibrous bump over the cut ends of the vas, or the two ends of the vas may join up again.

About one-third of men who have had vasectomy develop antibodies to sperm. The sperm go on being made but, unable to get past the blockage in the vas, they gradually deteriorate and then dissolve. The antibodies help in this process but whether that has any other effect is unknown. There is no evidence that these antibodies have any harmful consequences for men, although animal tests have occasionally shown hardening of the arteries in their blood vessels which might be linked to the antibodies.

Effectiveness

Because sperm take several months to be produced and to develop, there are always thousands of millions of them at various stages in the man's genital system. By cutting the vas, you stop new ones going right through the system, but you won't stop the ones which are past the break in the vas. Every time you ejaculate, you will get rid of some of these, until none are left.

You will therefore be asked to have occasional sperm-counts. How often you go depends on your individual doctor – some say that you should have one done after one, two, and three months; others after two or three months and not again unless there are a lot of sperm in the semen.

You will need to take along a freshly collected sample of your semen, either masturbated into a clean container, or in a recently used condom. Usually you will be told after two sperm-free tests that you can consider yourself no longer fertile. You may have to have additional counts if the sperm are slow to disappear, and if they don't disappear the vasectomy may have failed, which it occasionally can, perhaps because the vas has rejoined.

You will need to use another method of contraception until there have been two clear sperm counts. After that the risk of causing pregnancy is virtually nil.

Availability

Vasectomy is available under the National Health Service, free of charge. You may be referred to a hospital or a clinic by your family practitioner, or you may make an appointment at a family planning clinic, or your family practitioner may do the operation himself (quite a number of GPs are trained in vasectomy.) Even if your own doctor is not particularly enthusiastic, as you do not need his referral it is easier to get a vasectomy than female sterilisation.

More difficult is the question of how promptly you can get it. Waiting lists in different areas of the country vary from a few days to several months at hospitals and family planning vasectomy clinics. If you are in an area with a long waiting list, you may decide to have the operation done privately. Your doctor may be able to tell you if this is possible near where you live; alternatively the Margaret Pyke Centre and the Marie Stopes Clinic – both in London – offer an inexpensive service (see page 144 for both their addresses). The cost, including the follow-up sperm tests, should be under £60.

Most doctors will want to talk to you and be certain that you have understood that the operation can't be reversed, and that you are certain about what you are doing. Some still want a gap between their talk with you and the operation itself, to give you time to think it over – this may be a month or more.

You may find more difficulty in getting a vasectomy on the NHS if you are still in your 20s – even if you have completed your family – and especially if you have no children at all. This will vary from doctor to doctor, and, to some extent, on how articulate and determined you are. Again, if you have the operation done privately you are less likely to encounter opposition.

Some doctors like to talk to both partners before agreeing to do a vasectomy, on the grounds that this is an important decision which may lead to friction or unhappiness if it is not wanted by both the people involved. With a happy and mutually concerned couple, that is probably only commonsense. It does not have any legal basis, though – your partner does not have to sign a consent form before you have the operation – and if you have good reasons for wanting to keep the decision to yourself you should say so and insist on doing so.

Vasectomy is a simpler operation than female sterilisation, and is virtually free of long-term effects. Although most are done under a local anaesthetic, and therefore don't carry the hazards of a general anaesthetic, if you can't bear the idea of being conscious and if there are no particular personal health reasons for you to avoid one, your doctor may be willing to give you a general anaesthetic.

Once the tiny cuts have healed, it is effectively invisible. While this is generally an advantage, it can mean that a girl you don't know all that well may refuse to believe that you have had a vasectomy, and insist on using – or asking you to use – an additional contraceptive method. (There are ties, tie-pins, and so on, to show you have been vasectomised. Their motif is the scientific symbol for a male, with a small piece missing from the circle. But anybody can buy one . . .)

Having a vasectomy avoids the need ever to think about contraception again. It does not interfere with your sex-life or your masculinity, though if you were ambivalent about having it done your dislike of being totally infertile could affect your interest in sex. Although quite often the vas can be rejoined, and sperm may even appear in the semen, antibodies may prevent them fertilising an egg. You must assume vasectomy is permanent.

It has one potential drawback which is that if your partner later did become pregnant it would be very easy to tell whether the baby could be yours. A sperm test would reveal whether or not your vas had rejoined. If it had not, the consequences of knowing absolutely definitely that the pregnancy had nothing to do with you could be serious for both of you, and for any existing family.

Once you have decided that your family is complete, or that you will never want children in any circumstances, vasectomy, like female sterilisation, is probably one of the best methods of contraception. Given that most of the other methods are for women, many men consider that vasectomy offers them a chance to share the responsibility of avoiding pregnancy, and relieve their partner of the potential problems associated with other methods. But if you have been pressurised into it, you may well regret it later.

But this is only true if you have decided not just in your present circumstances but for the future too that you will not want children. If you have any feeling that a marriage is not a marriage without children, you should think very carefully about how a vasectomy might affect a future marriage. After all, however happy you are now, divorce is statistically not unlikely. What would you feel like if a future wife or partner wanted a family? If your existing children died in a fire or a car crash, say, would you be prepared to live without a family?

Some men, like some women, are just not interested in having children at all, and contraception has helped to make this a genuine and acceptable option. But if you don't think you will ever want children, again ask yourself if this is going to hold true for all time, whomever you meet, whatever pattern your life takes. The vast majority of men who have a vasectomy are pleased by the outcome and happy never to have to worry about causing an unintended pregnancy. But for a small minority it can be bitterly regretted.

Female sterilisation

There are a number of different ways in which a sterilisation operation can be done, but all of them involve the same basic idea, which is to block the Fallopian tubes so that the egg cannot be fertilised by sperm. The ovaries are not touched, so you go on having normal menstrual cycles until your natural menopause. When an egg is released each month, it simply travels down the tube as far as it can, then dies and gradually dissolves.

In some countries – particularly in the United States – women may be sterilised by having a hysterectomy (the removal of the womb). It is argued that as a few women later get cancer of the cervix, or of the lining of the womb, you might just as well have everything removed and avoid any later cancer risk. But hysterectomy is a major operation and like any major operation carries its own risks, including death, and we do not recommend that you choose it for sterilisation alone. If you have some additional medical condition your doctor may recommend hysterectomy, but that is quite a different matter.

Whichever method of sterilisation is used, there are some basic points which are common to all of them. None of the methods will affect your menstrual cycle or your sex life. A small number of women get heavier periods after sterilisation. Occasionally the stump of a tube may develop a small opening, or the tubes may grow together again. This is more common with some techniques than with others, but it is always a possibility. If it happens, you may get pregnant, and between 10–20 per cent of such pregnancies turn out to be ectopic.

If you think you want to be sterilised, you should be absolutely certain that whatever happens in the future you will not want another child. Depending on which technique is used, it might be possible if you changed your mind later to rejoin the tubes, but such operations are complicated and not always successful: there is no guarantee that even then you would get pregnant. The original sterilisation may simply have damaged the tubes too much for them to be put together again. Some doctors have had success rates of up to 70 per cent when they have rejoined tubes for women who had been sterilised by a method leaving the best hope for reversal. Even that, though, only gives you a two to one possibility of getting pregnant. The average rate of successful reversal is much lower. So you must assume that sterilisation is permanent.

Different types of sterilisation

Laparotomy This is often known as tubal ligation, or 'having my tubes tied'. It is not as serious an operation as, say, having your appendix out, but it does involve a general anaesthetic and a stay of a couple of days in hospital. A small cut is made (two or three inches in length) across your abdomen, usually just below the pubic hairline, though it may be higher if you have the operation at the same time as a baby or an abortion.

Then the surgeon brings the tubes to the surface, ties each tube in two places, and removes the small length in between the two ties. (There are a number of variations on this basic method: each surgeon has his own preferences. Tubes may be blocked with clips or bands, and the length to be removed may be crushed or burned – diathermy – instead of cut.)

You are likely to feel fairly uncomfortable for a day or two – as is the case with any operation which involves a cut across the abdomen – and you will probably need to take things easily for a few weeks.

Minilaparotomy This is not very different to a laparotomy, but the incision is shorter. A narrow speculum is inserted into the cut, so that the surgeon can see what he is doing. A special instrument is inserted into the womb from the vagina so that an assistant can push the womb and tubes towards the opening in the abdomen. It is not uncommon for a minilaparotomy to be done using a local anaesthetic, as an outpatient procedure; you may also feel less discomfort after the operation.

Female sterilisation

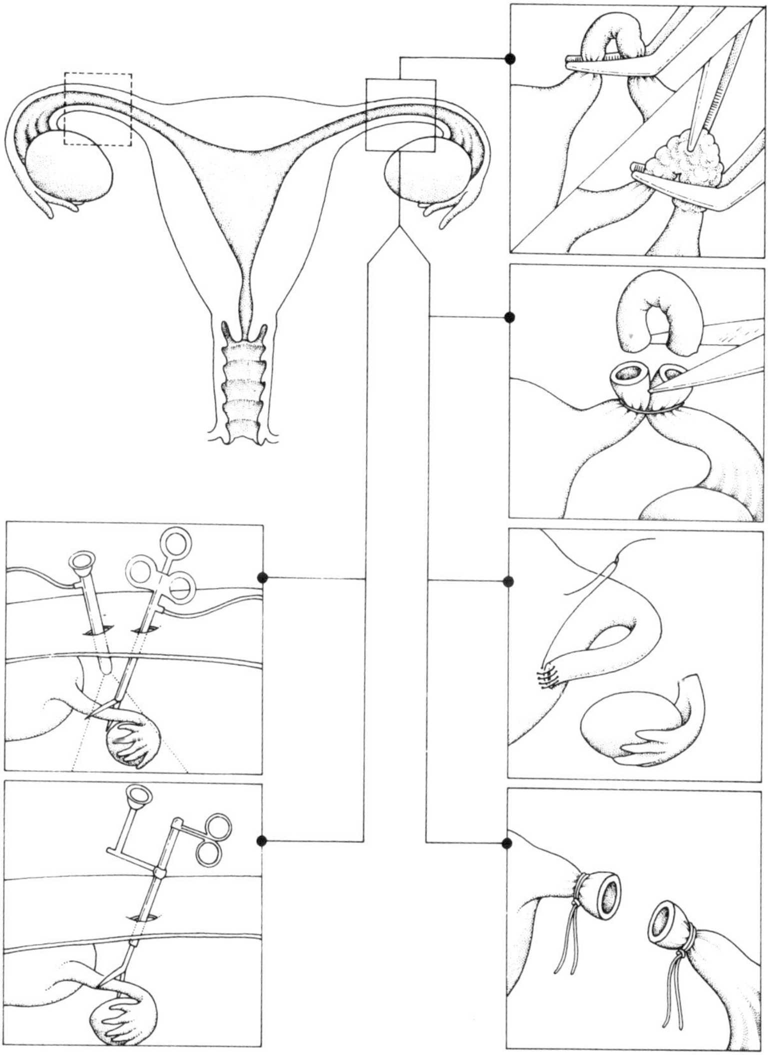

Laparoscopy techniques

Methods of occlusion of the Fallopian tubes

Laparoscopy A laparoscope looks like a very narrow telescope. It has tiny lenses which enable the surgeon to see your abdominal organs. Laparoscopes are used in all sorts of ways – often simply to help in diagnosing what is wrong with you – but some of them now incorporate instruments for putting silicon rubber bands or clips on the tubes to block them. More often the instrument that does the sterilisation is inserted through a second small incision. The laparoscope is always inserted through a cut (a mere half-inch long) just below the navel and the second incision made lower down, to one side. The operation is much the quickest and simplest of the various types of sterilisation as well as the least uncomfortable. It is easily done under a local anaesthetic, though some women prefer a general, and some doctors may prefer to give one.

Vaginal sterilisation Although the scars from a laparoscopy are almost invisible once they have healed, and the scars from the other types of sterilisation, if the cut has been made just below the pubic hairline, are pretty unnoticeable after they fade, some women prefer to have no visible scar. It is possible to do a sterilisation through the vagina instead, although the particular way the tubes are dealt with if you reach them this way means that it would be quite impossible even to attempt to rejoin them later. The operation is usually done under a general anaesthetic and if you have a vaginal sterilisation you must be particularly careful not to have sex until the time when your doctor says you can, otherwise you may not heal properly.

This operation is impossible if you have just had a baby or an abortion at more than 10 weeks' pregnancy because the tubes will be too far up to be reached. Vaginal sterilisations are not commonly done: they have the highest complication rates.

Safety

The side effects of sterilisation can be divided into those from a general anaesthetic, if you have one, and those from the operation itself. A general anaesthetic can make you feel quite ill, and it may lead to other side effects, like a lung infection, especially if you are a heavy smoker. But after all, thousands of people have them each year without any problems, so unless your doctor thinks that for some reason you would do better to avoid one, you should not worry. If he does think you should avoid having a general anaesthetic wherever possible, there are several types of sterilisation which can be done under a local anaesthetic.

The main group of complications with any sterilisation is from accidental damage to an organ or blood vessel near the tubes when the operation is being done. Many of these would be spotted and dealt with while the operation was still going on, but sometimes they are found in the few days afterwards. If you suffer bleeding, severe pain in the abdomen or womb, or a raised temperature, or have trouble urinating, you should see a doctor at once. All these complications are uncommon.

Because of the slightly increased risks of any operation if you are taking a combined Pill, you may be asked to stop taking it for a month, or perhaps even three months, before you are sterilised. (This also gives you a chance to get back to your normal periods, and check that they are indeed still normal.) You need of course to be very careful to use an alternative method of contraception during that time, to make sure you do not get pregnant in the interval.

There is some evidence that women who have been sterilised have heavier periods than others but it is not altogether clear whether this results from the sterilisation or is associated with other factors.

Effectiveness

Sterilisation is an extremely reliable way of ensuring you don't get pregnant: the failure rate is around 1 in 500 cases. In rare instances the tubes can rejoin by themselves, but this doesn't necessarily mean that they will do so in such a way that an egg can be fertilised.

Sometimes, the egg can get only part of the way down the tube but a sperm can reach it; if this happens you could have an ectopic pregnancy, so if you have sharp pains in the lower abdomen, especially with a missed period followed by slight vaginal bleeding, you should see a doctor.

Availability

You can get a sterilisation done under the National Health Service, but you must usually be referred to a hospital or to a gynaecologist by your family doctor. This can cause problems. Surveys indicate that, while the majority of doctors are quite happy to refer for sterilisation, some are less cooperative. They may consider you too young, or still feel that sterilisation is only suitable for women with more than five children, or they may just dislike the idea.

If your doctor is not helpful, there are several things you can do. One is to insist on your right to a second opinion and the chance to discuss the operation with a gynaecologist. You could try getting the name of doctors in your area who provide contraceptive advice for people other than their own patients (available from the local Family Practitioner Committee, libraries or post offices) and going to one of them. You could also see if your local family planning clinic can help.

Alternatively, you could decide to have the operation done privately. The Marie Stopes Clinic does sterilisations, at a cost of £99, plus £15 if you have a general anaesthetic; in both cases it is an out-patient operation where you go home after a few hours.

Most doctors, whether your GP or a gynaecologist, will want to talk to you and be sure that you have really understood that the operation can't be reversed and that you are certain about what you are doing. Some will want a gap between their first talk with you and the operation itself, to give you time to think it over – this may be a month or more.

You may find more difficulty getting sterilised on the NHS if you are very young (in your early 20s) even if you have completed a family, and especially if you have no children at all. Again, it varies from doctor to doctor and, to some extent, on how articulate and determined you are. In those circumstances you might want to consider having the operation done privately.

You might also want to go privately if there is a long waiting list for the operation in your area. In some local health authorities the wait may be as much as two years, which most people rightly find unacceptable. Just as your family doctor gets a special fee for providing family services, so too do those involved in hospital family planning services, such as sterilisation. In some areas this has increased their willingness to provide such services, but in others, once the money allocated on a rather arbitrary basis by the DHSS has been used up, no more sterilisations will be done until the end of the financial year.

Some doctors are keen to talk to both partners before sterilising one of them, on the grounds that this is an important decision which may lead to friction or unhappiness if it is not wanted by both the people involved. With a happy and mutually concerned couple, that is probably only commonsense. It does not have any legal basis though – a partner does not have to sign the consent form for the operation by law – and if you have good reasons for wanting to keep the decision to yourself you should say so and insist on it.

Acceptability

Sterilisation is a simple, minor operation. If you are afraid of any operation, you have the choice of either a general anaesthetic – in which case you won't see or know anything about it until it is all over – or a local one, when you are aware of everything being done to you, can talk to the doctor doing it, and climb off the couch afterwards by yourself; you may even walk out of the operating theatre.

It is extremely discreet – once the scars have faded they are so small that it is unlikely anybody will even notice them. It avoids the need for any kind of contraceptive appliance or having to think about contraception at all. It will not interfere with your sex life (unless you were ambivalent about having it done, in which case your dislike of being totally infertile could made you less interested in sex) and it should not affect your menstrual cycle.

It will keep you safe from pregnancy, usually without any long-term side effects and with only a tiny risk of immediate complications as a result of the operation.

Once you have decided that your family is complete, or that you will never want children in any circumstances, it is probably one of the best methods of contraception. But that is only true if you have made those decisions not just for now but for the future, too.

Studies show that a minority of women do later regret the operation – some, perhaps, because they came under pressure to have it done; others, because they hoped it might solve sexual or other marital problems (it won't); yet others, because their circumstances have later changed.

If you have any feeling that a marriage is not a marriage without children, you should think very carefully about how that might affect you in a future marriage. After all, however happy you are now, divorce is statistically not unlikely. If you married again, would you want his children? If he wanted children, how badly would you feel about not being able to have them? You need to think about whether, if your existing children died in a fire or a car crash, say, you would really be prepared to live without a family.

The existence of effective reversible contraception has made it easier for those women who are not interested in children to be able to avoid having them altogether, and a significant number now say openly that they will never have a family. But, again, you need to ask yourself, if you are one of these, if it is true for all time – even if you met a different man who wanted a family desperately, or later on, when you are established in your job (quite a number of women decide, at around the age of 30, that they do want children and had better have them at once before the risks of pregnancy start to increase with age).

The vast majority of women who are sterilised are delighted with the outcome, and find it a great relief to be able to forget the whole business of contraception, secure in the knowledge that they won't get pregnant. But for a small minority, it can be bitterly regretted.

New Horizons

New revolutionary contraceptives are regularly hailed by the media. They give new hope to people who don't like any of the existing methods, cause bafflement to their doctors when they go and ask for them, and then seem to disappear as mysteriously as they arrived.

So we thought we would include in this Guide a brief look at what might be available in the foreseeable future. Two things need to be stressed: first, there is nothing really revolutionary about any of them, and second, they are undergoing various sorts of animal and human tests and may or may not prove to be of much use.

There is little that is revolutionary, in the sense that the Pill was revolutionary – a totally new and different method of interfering with a different bit of the reproductive cycle, or in a different way. Most of the methods in this section are refinements of one or more of the contraceptives we've already described. They may be designed to reduce the side effects of a particular method, or make it easier to use, or more effective – but that is all.

One new idea, however, is the 'male Pill', discovered in China, and another is a contraceptive vaccine, but that only goes to prove another point – that if a new method is invented, there is so much research and testing to be done on it that by the time it might be available on general release, it will probably be too late to interest those of you who are reading this Guide in 1983. Inventing a drug is not half as difficult as testing it, ironing out as many snags as possible, retesting, and giving it clinical trials in humans. In the case of contraception, because you are a fit and healthy human being taking a contraceptive over a long period of time, the tests are even more stringent than for 'medical' discoveries – where the benefits of alleviating or possibly curing disease have to be weighed against any potential side effects. In the case of contraception, the whole process takes between 15 and 20 years.

Very few manufacturers are willing to tie up their investment over such a long period without any guarantee that the new contraceptive will ever get on to the market. International research, mainly carried out through the World Health Organisation, is only funded by a handful of governments and at a very low level. So the chances of a really new and infinitely better contraceptive within our reproductive lifetime are small.

Barriers

The renewed popularity of diaphragms and caps has led to new interest in improving them.

Small one-size diaphragm Tests are being carried out to see exactly what part the diaphragm plays in the diaphragm-and-spermicide contraceptive. If its only function is to hold the spermicide in place, then perhaps size is not so important and you wouldn't have to keep going to a doctor or clinic for a check. Alternatively, does the diaphragm block sperm even if it is not tightly fitted? In which case you could do away with the spermicide as well as with the repeat doctor's visits once you had been taught to use it.

Spermicide-impregnated diaphragm Like the new spermicide-impregnated condoms, this could be less of a chore and more acceptable (and therefore more reliable) than using a separate spermicide. Again, we won't really know how well they work until we establish how important the spermicide is, because it is not yet clear that spermicide-impregnated barriers are as reliable as barriers with additional separate spermicides.

Disposable diaphragms If it turns out that exact fitting of diaphragms is not all that important, disposable ones would offer the advantage of not having to be looked after. There would be no more worry about the rubber perishing, or a nail catching it, and no more careful washing and drying. You would simply go and buy a pack, like condoms, in one of a range of sizes – or perhaps even in a single size. Disposable diaphragms could also be made of biodegradable materials, to the relief of sanitary engineers.

Individualised cervical caps Caps could be more effective and more comfortable if they were moulded to the user's cervical shape. This is being done on the same principle that a dentist makes an impression of your mouth – the idea was in fact thought up by a dentist and a gynaecologist. The individualised cervical cap can have a one-way valve in it to allow menstrual fluid to escape, and in theory can be left in place for months. The recent discovery of a condition called 'toxic shock syndrome' in a few tampon-users in the United States has led to new concern about allowing secretions from the womb and the vagina to build up, so most authorities are not happy about the idea of leaving a cap in place for more than a few hours. There will have to be a lot more testing before we can be sure that the valve will eliminate any problems.

Vaginal rings These have been developed and can be made out of a variety of plastics and metals. They are a little like an IUD but fit into the cervical canal instead of the womb, and are therefore smaller. They can be impregnated with a long-acting spermicidal agent. It is still not clear exactly how they work or how effective and acceptable they are.

Collatex sponge Made of polyurethane foam, this is impregnated with a spermicide which acts by trapping sperm and blocking their path as well as by providing slow-release spermicide. It has a loop attached for removal, and is disposable. The version currently under trial is a modified one after earlier tests.

Collagen sponge Collagen is an extremely absorbent protein which makes it very effective at soaking up sperm. The sponge is also slightly acid, just like a healthy vagina, which means it has natural spermicidal qualities. Tests in Britain have just begun on a reusable collagen sponge.

Diaphragm/sponge One rather attractive idea has been to combine the virtues of both sponge and diaphragm, so that you get the absorbent capacity of the one with the better placing of the other. A device which looks rather like a powder-puff and is made of spongy collagen has a reinforced rim inside it, consisting of a flexible rubber ring. The sponge is impregnated with a spermicide and is disposable.

Tests have only just begun.

Diaphragms, sponges and caps in their new versions have many of the same plusses and minuses as their prototypes, as far as acceptability goes. They are likely to have a low incidence of side effects and to be fairly reliable. Some of the new ones sound as if they would be easier to use and therefore more likely to get regular use. They won't appeal to women who dislike handling their vulva and initial training at a clinic or by a doctor or nurse may still be needed, so that the woman is taught to identify her cervix and use the method properly.

Condoms Condom modifications are fairly minor, and involve testing thinner ones to see if their effectiveness can be kept but sensation improved; new synthetic materials are being used and biodegradable condoms researched (traditional ones don't break down and tend to block sewage plants, so cost a lot to deal with).

Hormonal contraceptives

LH-RH In the section on the Pill, we described the way the luteinising hormone triggers the reproductive cycle. It in turn is controlled by a chemical messenger produced by the pituitary – the *luteinising hormone-releasing hormone*, or LH-RH. It works both to induce and inhibit ovulation, depending on the dosage and the timing of the dose. This hormone has been synthesised and a more potent version of it produced. It also works in men by inhibiting the formation of sperm.

The interesting thing about LH-RH is that unlike the Pill it works only on very limited areas of the body. While oestrogens and progestagens affect all sorts of tissues, LH-RH acts only on the pituitary gland, the testis and the ovary. It also stops working within minutes of being used, and is rapidly broken down – again unlike the Pill. So it is theoretically a great deal safer, and less likely to produce a whole range of side effects.

Nasal spray Tests are going on in various countries using LH-RH or one of its derivatives in the form of a nasal spray which women can sniff. It is still not clear what the lowest effective dose is, and it seems that it would interfere with menstrual bleeding.

Single day LH-RH If LH-RH is given on one day in the second half of the menstrual cycle, it brings on menstruation. This single-day dose interferes less with the menstrual cycle, and with menstrual bleeding, but it is not yet known if it would actually prevent pregnancy – only that it does bring on a period in non-pregnant women. It could, possibly, be used as a once-a-month method.

The male nasal spray The same nasal spray idea, used on men, seems to cause a decrease in sex drive after a few weeks because the level of male hormones is reduced, although it also seems to inhibit sperm production. So as well as finding the lowest effective dose, research into adding androgens (male hormones) back in is being carried out – but it seems a complicated way of doing things.

Oestrogen/Progestagen

One drawback of the Pill is having to take it daily. A variety of long-acting versions of the Pill are being tested, or rather of the Pills, because some of them contain both an oestrogen and a progestagen while others are progestagen-only.

A monthly injection Instead of the three-monthly DMPA, a monthly injection helps to control the irregular bleeding which is associated with the existing injectable. In addition to the progestagen-only version, a combined monthly injection is also under trial.

Implants On the other hand, implants make it possible to provide a contraceptive which will last for up to five years, but which is removable if you decide you want to get pregnant. Very tiny capsules of silicone rubber are put under the skin. They are impregnated with contraceptive hormones which are released very gradually. If you change your mind, the process of removal is a little more complicated than having them implanted in the first place – but it is possible.

Another type of implant is to use biodegradable polymers, which disintegrate in the body. These allow for implants so small that they can be injected, and for varying doses to be given, so that you could in theory ask for anything from a month's supply to a couple of years'. When the polymers break down, though, they are absorbed into the body, so that there is still quite a lot of research to be done on whether this could be harmful.

Steroidal rings Rings and other devices impregnated with long-acting hormones have been designed to fit into the vagina. The hormones are absorbed into the bloodstream and work in the same way as the Pill. The ones which are progestagen-only carry the usual problems of breakthrough bleeding and interference with the menstrual cycle; those with an oestrogen as well cause much less interference, but nobody is yet sure what their long-term effects on the vagina and cervix could be. Vaginal rings have the advantage that you can insert and remove them yourself.

Steroidal IUDs With a conventional IUD, the problem is getting them large enough to work and not fall out, but not so large that you get pain and bleeding. By adding a long-acting hormone to the IUD, you should be able to get greater reliability from a much smaller device, and some advantages, such as lighter periods. Some of them don't even look much like a conventional IUD, being made of polymer fibres which can be arranged into almost any shape. Besides avoiding a number of the usual side effects of IUDs, hormonal IUDs may be a safer way to use hormones because they work directly on the lining of the womb and very little of their ingredients is released into the bloodstream. The same could be true of hormones placed in the cervix, but researchers are still having difficulty in discovering the best design for a cervical device which would carry the hormones.

The 'male Pill'

At the moment there are two possible male Pills around. The first sort has been described under LH-RH earlier in this section. The second sort was discovered by the Chinese, and is made from gossypol which is present in cotton seed. Trials in China have suggested that some of the men given gossypol for a long period have delays in becoming fertile again, and may never make as many sperm in the future. They have also found a decrease in blood potassium, which could be a serious ill-effect. The Chinese say that it is unlikely that a gossypol Pill would be cleared for general distribution for some years, and Western researchers on gossypol agree.

Prostaglandins

Prostaglandins are substances which influence the muscles in the womb, causing contractions. They are found naturally in both men and women, and are often given to induce a baby. For at least the past ten years, people have thought that prostaglandins would make an ideal once-a-month contraceptive, because they may prevent the fertilised egg from embedding itself in the womb's lining, as well as causing a very early abortion if one has been implanted. In theory, all you would have to do is take prostaglandins when your period was due, and it would arrive. In fact, though, prostaglandins have been one of the great contraceptive disappointments – a high dose is needed and it brings on painful cramps, diarrhoea and sickness. So far, prostaglandins seem more useful as a very early way of inducing menstruation, rather than as a regular contraceptive, despite much research over the last decade to improve the possibilities.

RU472

A steroid has been discovered which interferes with the body's progesterone and interrupts the phase of the cycle when the egg is released. This suggests that it could be a useful contraceptive but it is still at a very early stage.

Identifying ovulation

As we said in the section on Periodic Abstinence, there are all sorts of changes in your body around the time of ovulation. The more of those changes you can measure, the nearer you are likely to be to a method which will not only pinpoint ovulation but – more difficult – predict it.

This would cut down considerably the time during which you would have to avoid sex if you were not using another contraceptive. Research into measuring the hormonal content of your urine, with a kit which changes colour according to the urine's chemical changes, is quite far advanced. So too are a variety of microchip computers which can measure several symptoms at the same time, like temperature, changes in your sweat and saliva. Some of the gadgets are designed to be worn, such as a bracelet or pendant; others are larger. At the moment, all of them are better at measuring when you do ovulate than at telling you at least five days in advance that you will do – and that is very important if you want to have sex in the first half of the cycle. In fact, it is still so difficult to predict how long sperm will survive that if a woman doesn't want to become pregnant she is going to have to continue to avoid sex altogether except in the second half of the cycle.

Vaccines

Vaccines are the other really innovative area of contraceptive research. The most advanced is probably a vaccine against human chorionic gonadotrophin (hCG) which is a hormone essential for maintaining pregnancy. Human trials are to begin shortly, but there is a lot still to be discovered about the effectiveness and how long this would last in humans. Other vaccines being developed include one which would affect a specific sperm enzyme, and another which would affect the zona pellucida (which surrounds the egg), through which sperm have to penetrate to fertilise the egg.

Abortion

There are two basic kinds of abortion: spontaneous and induced. About 15 per cent of all pregnancies end in a miscarriage (spontaneous abortion), many of them so early on that you don't even know you have been pregnant.

The other sort of abortion is induced. It can be carried out deliberately and legally for several different reasons: if there is a real risk of the baby being born handicapped; or because continuing the pregnancy would affect your physical or mental health or the physical or mental health of your existing children; or where your life is put at risk by continuing the pregnancy.

In England and Wales, the 1967 Abortion Act does not say that you can have an abortion simply because you want one. In Scotland, the law is slightly different but in practice works like it does in England. In Northern Ireland, the law remained unchanged in 1967 and is much more strict: generally, abortion is only available if there is a serious risk to your life as a result of the pregnancy (that is why many women come to England from Northern Ireland to have an abortion).

Up to twelve weeks of pregnancy, the most common way to carry out an abortion is by suction. A narrow flexible polythene tube is slid into your womb through the cervix and the contents are removed using a suction pump. If you are only a few weeks' pregnant, it may not even be necessary to widen the cervix in order to slide the tube up; after the first month or so the cervix will have to be stretched gently and gradually to allow a larger tube to pass through.

These suction abortions (vacuum aspiration, as they are often called) can be done under a local or a general anaesthetic. Some doctors give you a choice. There is a certain risk in having any general anaesthetic, so it is usually a good thing to avoid wherever possible. It can be done as an out-patient procedure so that you can go home the same day, but unfortunately there are only about 17 day-care abortion centres around the country under the NHS, so unless you are lucky enough to have one close to you, an

NHS abortion will probably involve an overnight stay. (On the one hand doctors complain that abortions clutter up hospital beds which could more usefully be used for other things; on the other they are doing remarkably little to reduce that bed-load by alternatives like day-care surgery.)

Suction abortion is much the safest way of performing an abortion, for several reasons. Not only can it be done with a local anaesthetic, but the flexible tube is very unlikely to do any damage to your womb or your cervix, and there is very little blood loss. However, many women get quite severe cramps while the procedure is being carried out, so a general anaesthetic is still popular.

After about 12 weeks abortion is more usually done by *dilatation and curettage* (D and C). This means dilating, or stretching, the cervix and removing the contents of the womb with metal instruments. It is done under a general anaesthetic and involves an overnight stay. There is a small risk of the metal instruments perforating the womb, or causing damage to the cervix or the bladder, and there is greater blood loss.

Alternatives to a D and C later in the pregnancy are injections into the womb of various substances, like prostaglandins or saline, which cause the womb to contract and the foetus to be expelled. The injections usually lead to an abortion within 12–36 hours, but they often have to be followed by curettage to empty the womb completely, because the placenta may be left behind. The waiting period can be very distressing, and the actual abortion involves contractions like labour pains.

An alternative to prostaglandin injections is *dilatation and evacuation* (D and E) which is carried out under a general anaesthetic and needs an expert surgeon. In very rare cases, you may have to have a hysterotomy. (This should not be confused with hysterectomy, which is removing the womb.) Hysterotomy is rather like having a caesarean birth, with a stomach operation to remove the foetus, and is of course done under a general anaesthetic. It leaves a scar on the womb, as well as a visible one on your abdomen, which could cause complications if you had a later pregnancy. You should seek a second opinion if this operation is suggested without a good medical reason, such as cervical fibroids.

Safety

There is one absolutely vital thing to remember about abortion – the earlier it is done the safer it is. This applies regardless of the methods, the skills of individual surgeons or whatever else has been measured. A study in the United States showed that if you have an abortion at under eight weeks' pregnancy, the chances of death are 1 for every 100,000 abortions. At 16 to 20 weeks, that chance goes up to 24 deaths for every 100,000 abortions, and at 21 weeks or over the risk is more than 34 deaths.

It is essential that if you think you could be pregnant, but are too late to use post-coital contraception, you should move quickly if you want to get an abortion (see the section on availability).

Besides being safer in the sense that you are much less likely to die from it, early abortion by vacuum aspiration carries fewer immediate or long-term risks. You don't have the dangers to the cervix or womb that using metal instruments involves, and there is no evidence that the abortion will have any more effect on a later pregnancy than a spontaneous abortion does. (There seems to be a slightly higher chance of premature labour, low birth-weight and even spontaneous abortion in the fourth to sixth months of a following pregnancy if you have a D and C, perhaps because of slight damage to the cervix.)

Emotionally, too, an early abortion is much less traumatic than a later one, especially if that later one is done by injection into the womb so that it takes time and involves labour pains and a delivery through the vagina. There is no evidence that physically and mentally healthy women suffer any severe emotional effects after having an abortion, if that is what they wanted.

Obviously, if you did not want an abortion, but decided to have one – perhaps because there was a serious risk of the baby being deformed – you may have more difficulty in accepting the loss. And if you are not sure whether or not you really want an abortion, you need to think about and talk to someone about the decision very carefully and thoroughly before you finally make up your mind.

Abortion and sterilisation

Whichever type of abortion you have, it always carries a higher risk if it is done at the same time as sterilisation. This means that unless there are good medical or personal reasons for you to have the two done together, you should avoid a double operation.

Some doctors have been known to imply – or even to say directly – that they will only let you have an abortion if you will agree to be sterilised at the same time. There is no legal – or other – justification for this and you should not be pressurised into accepting. Sterilisation is a serious long-term decision which cannot be made a condition for abortion. If your doctor tries to make any such suggestion, go elsewhere.

Availability

Getting an abortion is not always easy and it varies a lot round the country. All we can do here is give some general guidelines and emphasise again that speed is essential – don't allow yourself to be put off or stalled if you are certain of what you want.

Unless you have some very good reason for not talking to your doctor about it, you should go and see him immediately you think you are pregnant. He will probably do a pregnancy test but if he says the results will take several days you may want to get one done elsewhere to save time. You should explain to your doctor exactly why you don't want to have the baby, and the problems you foresee both for yourself and your family if you have one.

If your doctor refuses to help you, ask him why. It may

be that he genuinely feels that you do not qualify for an abortion under the Abortion Act. Or he may be affected by his religious views or his conscience. If he is refusing because of religion or conscience, don't get angry – he is entitled to, both legally and morally. But he should refer you to a colleague who will advise you. You can ask him to do this. Some doctors don't go as far as actually refusing to refer you, but try to delay matters to give you more time to get accustomed to the idea of pregnancy. You may be asked to come back after a few weeks to see whether you have missed a second period or not. If you have made up your mind about an abortion, don't wait; ask him to refer you immediately, or go elsewhere. A family planning clinic doctor may be helpful.

As far as contraception in general is concerned, we have said that you can always try another GP in your area for contraceptive services which your own GP won't provide. In the case of abortion, although the same applies in theory, it probably won't work in practice. For one thing, a GP who does not know you may be hesitant about referring you for an abortion; for another, finding an alternative will just take too long. You will probably have to go to one of the charitable abortion services (see below).

However, assuming for the moment that you have an understanding and sympathetic doctor, his next step after seeing you is to refer you to a hospital doctor. He has to agree that you qualify for an abortion under the Act, and that he or his staff will actually do it.

This is where the next delay can arise. The hospital staff may not notice that you want an appointment for an abortion, so give you a date several weeks ahead. Or your nearest hospital may be very booked up and genuinely unable to offer you an appointment for some time. Or the consultant may be another believer in the value of stalling. If you can't get an appointment quickly, check with the appointments staff to make sure they know why you want it, and if you have no luck, go back to your doctor and ask him to refer you to another hospital in the area where there is a shorter waiting list.

If you can't get a hospital appointment quickly, you may have to go outside the NHS.

There are several registered charities who carry out abortions: the biggest are the Pregnancy Advisory Service (in London) and the British Pregnancy Advisory Service, which has fourteen centres around the country. They offer pregnancy testing, and will interview you and examine you to decide whether you are eligible for an abortion, as well as performing the operation in their own clinics. You do not have to be referred by your GP – though many women are – and they have a helpful counselling service so that if you haven't entirely made up your mind whether or not you want an abortion they will help you to discuss all the issues and possible options.

The surveys suggest that counselling can be useful for some women, though many have made up their minds before they ever get to see a doctor. If you feel you do want to discuss the question, make sure you are given the opportunity to talk to a counsellor.

One problem is that the counsellors may not be seen as independent advisers, but as part of the group making the decision over whether or not you will get your abortion. It can seem difficult to raise any doubts with a counsellor who is seeing you before or after the consultant considers your request, but you should take the opportunity to express your feelings. And the fact that your GP has referred you doesn't automatically mean that your request will be granted. Some GPs pass on women to the hospital because they are reluctant to spoil their relationship with a patient by saying 'no', but hope the consultant will. Others simply have a more liberal view on abortion than the consultant may have.

The final delay may indeed arise at the consultant stage. Some hospitals can offer you an abortion within a few days from your first appointment. Others may only offer you a date for the operation which is some weeks ahead. The faster you have been able to get through the previous hurdles, the more likely you are now to have a little time in hand, in case it is needed. Worst of all, the consultant may refuse to agree that you are eligible for an abortion, and you will have to start all over again . . .

Fewer than half the women in Britain who want an abortion get one on the NHS, but don't despair. Most of the rest go to the charities who try to keep their costs as low as possible, and who will try to help you with an interest-free loan if you are really unable to pay. (Even bank managers now accept that their customers may need a loan for an abortion!)

The major drawback to the charities, as far as availability goes, is that if you live outside one of the major cities, they are not so easy to get to as your local hospital. Set against that, they are often able to do the whole thing – counselling and abortion – within a couple of days, which may be more convenient than a hospital. And they can offer day care if you live nearby.

There are also some commercial abortion agencies. These acquired a bad name in the late 1960s and early 1970s when some of them touted for business, using taxi-drivers to sweep up bewildered foreigners at London Airport, and charged inflated prices for what was often an inadequate service. Nowadays they are more strictly controlled by the Department of Health and Social Security, and many of them offer a perfectly good service. Their prices have also come down but are still higher than the charitable sector, so unless you are fanatical about private medicine, they are not really a good idea.

Acceptability

Nobody much likes the idea of abortion, and certainly it is not an alternative to contraception. But, as there is no perfectly reliable contraceptive, accidental pregnancies will continue to happen. What you feel about abortion will depend on your individual principles, upbringing and beliefs – but most women can think of at least some circumstances in which it might be the best option.

All we can say here is that very early abortion is always preferable to later abortion: safer, and generally less upsetting. The law, though, is very much a question of interpretation and, in general, women wanting an abortion find the series of hurdles involved in getting it the worst part about it. You may have to be very determined and prepared to argue with receptionists, GPs and consultants, or to traipse around the country finding a charitable service. You have to refuse to accept delays, and refuse to take no for an answer. The importance of quick action is getting through, though, and each year the proportion of abortions done at under 12 weeks rises, as both doctors and the women involved become aware of the need for speed.

Menstrual regulation

A suction abortion can be carried out even if you don't know definitely that you are pregnant. It is done within two weeks of missing a period. Some trials were done in Britain in which women whose periods were late underwent vacuum aspiration. This removes the lining of the womb which would come away if you were having your period; it wouldn't necessarily include a fertilised egg.

When it is done as early as this, the tube can be slipped through the cervix without any stretching, and even without a local anaesthetic. Some people have argued that you could have this done each month as a method of contraception, and it would solve the moral dilemma for some women which an actual abortion – knowing they are pregnant – involves.

But enough women in the trials found it uncomfortable enough for it to become clear that routine menstrual regulation was not really an appropriate contraceptive alternative.

It also counts under English law as an abortion technique, so that trial centres wanting to do it had to be licensed in the same way and conform to all the legal procedures, such as getting two doctors to agree before you could have it done. Although it is a very safe procedure, doctors were also a bit reluctant to keep inserting an instrument into the womb, perhaps unnecessarily.

Nowadays you have to wait until after a pregnancy test shows that you really are pregnant before you go for menstrual regulation. (There is a new pregnancy test you can have before you miss a period.)

Illegal abortion

If you are tempted to think that one way around the hurdles of getting a legal abortion is to try it some other way – don't! Before the 1967 Abortion Act there were an estimated 60–100,000 illegal abortions each year. Many of these left the woman in hospital with severe infection or permanent damage to the womb. Many others resulted in the woman's death.

There is no safe and reliable way of causing an abortion at home. Most of the folk methods either don't have any effect at all, or are likely to kill you. Things like alcohol or quinine won't work unless you take a dose which will poison or kill you. Implements pushed up into the womb will kill or injure you or cause infection; syringes full of soapy water or antiseptic may do the same.

An attempted back-street abortion of these kinds can, if it doesn't injure or kill you, leave a live but deformed foetus. It also carries a maximum penalty of life imprisonment.

The only safe abortion is a legal abortion.

Appendices

Measuring the effectiveness of contraceptives

There are several different ways which researchers use to measure how well contraceptives work.

Theoretical, or method effectiveness

This takes into account only those pregnancies which occur when the technique is used regularly and correctly. If, for example, anybody admits to having taken a Pill late, or used a cap without spermicide in an emergency, any pregnancy which results is not included in the total. Only those pregnancies which are directly due to the failure of the method used correctly are included. As a result, 'theoretical effectiveness' is an estimate of the best possible results under ideal circumstances.

Classical use-effectiveness

This includes pregnancies which occur when the method is used regularly, though not necessarily in the correct way. So if you got pregnant while using a cap, that pregnancy would count towards the failure rate, but those doing the study would check to see if you had always used the cap properly. If you had, it would count as 'method failure', and if you had not, it would go down as 'user failure'.

Extended use-effectiveness

This includes in the failure rate all pregnancies which happen during the course of the research, whether or not the method is used correctly and regularly. Only couples who withdraw from the study, either to have a baby or to change methods, are excluded from the results.

Each technique has pros and cons. *Method effectiveness* tells you what is potentially possible in the way of reliable contraception, if you are absolutely robot-like in your efficiency in using it. *Classical use-effectiveness*, which is the most widely used method of evaluating contraceptive efficiency, gives some idea of how easy or difficult a method is to use – for instance, if the method failure is 2 for every 100 woman-years, but the user rate is 7, there is clearly quite a lot of scope for a slip-up. The most 'realistic' in some ways is *extended use-effectiveness*, which does not bother with the rather arbitrary distinctions in classical use-effectiveness but simply says that in a particular population your chances of getting pregnant with such and such a method are x per hundred women per year. The snag with this one is that groups being tested vary a lot, and the rate from a study containing extremely keen and conscientious women may not be remotely like another obtained elsewhere.

Whichever measure is used, the risks of pregnancy are summed up either using what is called the Pearl Index, or with a life-table formula. The Pearl Index simply takes the number of users and the number of months they used the method and calculates the pregnancies for every hundred women for a year. This is expressed in terms of failures per hundred woman-years or user-years. This is the traditional measurement, but it does not take into account that most contraceptives have a higher failure rate in the first year, until the users have settled down with the method, or until those who weren't keen on the method have dropped it.

So a lot of recent studies of contraceptives use life-tables, which do show pregnancies over time, and the users who drop out of the study, in far more detail. Unfortunately life-table analysis is far more difficult for the non-statistician to grapple with, although it is certainly a better method of evaluation.

As you can see from the different ways of measuring effectiveness, and from the different ways of summarising the information, the results can also be pretty varied. This is why we have not used any absolute figures for the failure rates of different contraceptives: it depends too much on what you are measuring and in what circumstances.

Questions to ask about contraceptive studies

A large number of contraceptive studies are reported in the press. These are some of the questions you may wish to ask when trying to decide how important the findings are.

1. How many women or men were involved, and over what period of time?

2. How recent are the findings? (The fact that they are newly published does not necessarily mean that the study has only just been completed: it may be a re-analysis of a much older study, for example, which looked at contraceptives now outdated.)

3. Do the reports specify exactly which brands, doses or types of the contraceptive were studied?

4. Are the risks of use, or the efficiency of the method, discussed in relation to the age of the user?

5. In the case of risks, does the study take other factors into account, like predisposing medical problems, number of partners, etc?

6. Is the study prospective – looking at the population as time goes by and seeing what conditions crop up, or retrospective – noticing that x women who have come up with a particular problem all used the same contraceptive?

7. When possible, consider the source – who financed the study and is any group's self-interest involved?

Addresses

British Pregnancy Advisory Service
2nd Floor
58 Petty France
Victoria
London SW1

01-222 0985

Brook Advisory Service
153A East Street
London SE17

01-708 1234

Family Planning Information Service
27-35 Mortimer Street
London W1

01-636 7866

Marie Stopes House
Well Woman Centre
108 Whitfield Street
London W1

01-388 0662

Pregnancy Advisory Service
11-13 Charlotte Street
London W1

01-637 8962

Margaret Pyke Centre
15 Bateman Buildings
Soho Square
London W1

01-734 9351

Natural Family Planning Service
Catholic Marriage Advisory Council
15 Lansdowne Road
London W11

01-727 0141

Natural Family Planning Unit
Birmingham Maternity Unit
Queen Elizabeth Medical Centre
Edgbaston
Birmingham 15

021-472 1377 (ext. 102)